A SILENT
STRONG MAN

A man suffers from the most deadly illness in the latter stage of his life turning out gaining a precious and touching experience with his four children. For all they lose—those four children have learned a substantial lesson—despite bitter, teaching them never love too late that will be definitely influential and beneficial to their lives afterwards.

A SILENT
STRONG MAN

Never Love Too Late!

Judy Cheng

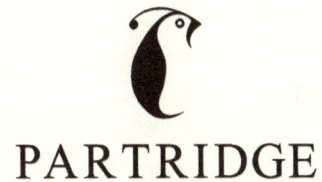

PARTRIDGE

ISBN: Hardcover   978-1-4828-2784-2
             Softcover   978-1-4828-2783-5
             eBook   978-1-4828-2785-9

To order additional copies of this book, contact
Toll Free +65 3165 7531 (Singapore)
Toll Free +60 3 3099 4412 (Malaysia)
orders.singapore@partridgepublishing.com

www.partridgepublishing.com/singapore

For
My sister, May Cheng

And for my two brothers, Samuel Cheng and John Cheng

Especially for my sons, Tommy and Simon, mainly
because I want to let them know something special inside
their grandpa—whom they have never known before

PREFACE

I write the book mainly for the remembrance of my father, who, through his whole life, had unwittingly given us an image that he did not need love. Not until he was heavily laden with a deadly illness, long lying in bed and staying at the hospital, did we unexpectedly find him an affectionate person who liked talking and needed love. What a pity—such a false image he had all along projected, making us love him far, far less.

My very aim of writing this book is to share with people my experiences and to alert all the people who have fathers to immediately talk to them and love them, especially when they— inexplicably, usually—find them so silent and strong that they seem unlikely to need love. As to the side of fathers—who, most of the time, tend to display their strongest to their children while attempting to build up a father's icon in a family—I hope they will not only let their children know they need their children's love but also allow themselves to love after receiving the message of the book.

CHAPTER ONE

Today, 2012 Father's Day, we would be going to celebrate it in an unusual way and mood—Father is staying at the hospital, expecting to receive a substantial and dangerous surgery the day after tomorrow.

This being, ever in our lives, the most special Father's Day, we all went see Father with laughter and joy on the surface, worries and sadness beneath. Impressively, Father was sitting on the bed with a not bad countenance, waving to us when we arrived. Seeing him acting so positive and optimistic, we, in a way, were a little more relieved when we were very much worried earlier. However, we knew we needed a lot more than relief—that was, we had to give Father as much *support* and *love* as possible to help create a miracle for him the day after tomorrow to survive the surgery. There were no two ways about it.

With that, we chatted with Father freely with casual topics, hoping at least he would not find out we were so much worried and anxious deep down. In the meantime, we could not but find this kind of pretence—despite being one so flimsy as to easily be seen through—a useful tool on which we now greatly depended. Father, too, knew how to employ such pretence, talking with us as if the day after tomorrow was nothing but a normal day. He chose not to talk about the operation, nor did he talk any about the pain stemming from the preparations he was taking now—the laxative prescription.

Nevertheless, when we saw him taking the laxative the doctor prescribed him with a purpose of forcing him to have a full excretion to clear all the solid wastes from his bowels before the surgery that he would take, there was an immediate emotional toll on us despite Father not showing us a bit of pain on his face. Surprisingly, he talked with us with not a little humour, recalling many memories of yore to prepare more subjects for us to talk with.

He showed us a shaver we four siblings sent him as his birthday present three decades ago, saying it was the best shaver in the world to make him keep using today. At once, the good old days, when we were young and living together, were conjured up memories in our minds like a review. We remembered that we had used the money (which we scraped up each day) from our cash box to buy Father that shaver when we were still students. Father must have treasured it as pearl, or he would not have kept using it. Awesomely, he kept that shaver so well that it could look like a new one, defying age. Father was an exceedingly grateful person, and 'Waste not, want not' was an axiom he had shown in many cases in his life.

An hour passed by. Father signalled us to leave with a series of movements, from getting up of the bed to heading the washroom. We knew it was the effect of the laxative he was prescribed. Before we said goodbye to him, he asked us not to come tomorrow, saying he would be busier and unable to entertain us. Father was elite in employing sardonic humour. We laughed, grasping what he meant. We waved him goodbye, promising him we would come early the day after tomorrow morning, before he would be into the operation room. Father, again, appeared with a countenance of peacefulness and just nodded with a slight and sweet smile.

Father was diagnosed with the *terminal* stage of colon cancer.

Unrivalled in its brutality, illness has inevitably played a significant role in our lives, making us unable to flee but ready to face with courage.

The coming days would definitely be arduous and grim for Father. However much arduous and grim those were, we promised with each other that we would be by Father's side to fight the battle with him with gritty resolve until the end. As amazing as life can be, it is not always beer and skittles. There are times when it is bitter black coffee. Only those who grasp the way to taste it will earnestly realize the wonderfulness and true meaning of life.

What life literally tells us is we are born surviving adventures, with the very first chapter of the way we come into the world as a clear proof.

With the evening approaching, I appeared so laden that David, my husband, found it imperative to console me. 'Don't be too worried. Everything will be fine. Worry doesn't work.' He gently said to me. With that, everything went forward as usual—dinner, television, and then going to sleep. Conceivably, I hardly slept one wink, spending the whole night asking all the gods I could name to bless Father. It seemed to be good for me when I lay total awake the whole night, for I got up on time without fail. Although there was more than enough time for us to go to the hospital, all the same, I felt we had to rush, fearful that we would be late to miss the chance to see Father before he was into the operation room. Within ten minutes, David and I rushed downstairs to find transportation.

As soon as we got to Father, we saw him already fully prepared sitting on a wheelchair and heading to the operation room.

Father smiled saying good morning to us. We greeted him with love, eager to touch him but finding nowhere appropriate— he was already dressed, geared up for an operation with sanitary clothes and cap on his head. Not knowing what to say that would be right, we chose to smile, smile, and smile. At the last moment, we said to him from the bottom of our hearts, 'See you later!' Father replied to us with a big 'Yes!' Clearly, he was confident. Sam and John, my two younger brothers, were there too, suggesting a breakfast downstairs at the canteen. Our eldest sister, May, could not take a leave from school, being a teacher there. She said she would come in the afternoon. Our mother would come too, except without saying the time.

Truly, it was one of the biggest days ever in our lives.

Sam and John explained Father's situation to us while we were taking breakfast at the hospital's canteen. They said Dr Chu, one of the most prestigious doctors in Hong Kong specializing in curing the colon cancer, diagnosed Father in a rather mortal illness. The tumour inside Father's colon was so *big* that part of it had already implanted onto his bladder, making him frequently pee day and night. Dr Chu said that he would remove the part of the colon with the tumour and the bladder. He saw Father would stand a great possibility to survive the operation, and if the recovery could be as smooth as expected, he might have at least several years to live, on the condition that the cancer would not come back too quickly. He added it would still be a miracle for an octogenarian as Father if all the foregoing did happen. As to such miracle, it would rely much more on Father's will and his mental than his physical tenacity.

According to what Dr Chu said, we thought we had enough reasons to believe such miracle would happen to Father, with Father's strong willingness to live. Father was a person who knew what life was. 'Never expect and always satisfy' was his magical way to live. He could live in the simplest way, easily getting contented with small things. We cannot but conclude him a man hard to come by in a world of utilitarianism.

Two hours passed by. Mother arrived. She brought Father a pot of congee, saying he might want something to eat after the surgery. She might not know a patient cannot eat anything right after operation. She sat down saying how tired she was without asking much about Father's situation. Instead, she read the newspaper, talking some issues popular or unpopular with us, whiling away time.

'Dr Chu said the operation might take at least four hours to get done if it went smoothly,' John said, as if wanting to tell Mother about the time. To all intents and purposes, we had already talked about the details of Father's operation before. Mother responded with a seemingly startled expression plus a sigh before going on with her newspaper reading. Literally, she was exceedingly tired. As for us, we looked at our watches most of the time this morning, hoping Father could come out of the operation room within the said time Dr Chu reckoned.

Hours passed the slowest ever this morning when we were more than laden waiting.

We were not disappointed. Father came out of the operation room within the said time. At that very moment upon hearing the news informed by the nurse, we almost cried out.

From the word *go*, we immediately packed the stuff we left on the tables at the canteen and rushed upstairs by taking the lift to the room Father stayed. Although we perceivably knew we got the news that Father had come out, we still dared not believe it real. Such sentiment we had was so strong that it triggered much of our emotions, and such emotions was so overcome that we found ourselves stirred. The result was we rushed jostling our way to bump into others to take elevator to get to Father.

After a series of work and care done by the nurses, we could finally approach Father. The first sight we got of him was nothing but convulsing despite us thinking we were fully prepared to see what he was supposed to be. Seeing him lying in bed with several medical tubes respectively fixed to his nose, mouth, and hand, we could not but be shocked. We were shocked because we could not know if Father could stand the scale of devastation the operation done to him. We were shocked because we could not know if he could make the recovery. Still, we went through the motions of not acting scared by the scene with the flimsy pretence we had mastered lately, showing each other composure and confidence. Father was still plunged into unconsciousness, and we stood by his side, waiting and observing.

Minutes later, a nurse came to us with a plastic bag of something we had never ever seen in our lives. Clearly, she needed our attention to her. Without psychologically preparation, we were all startled as an immediate response. Given the circumstances, we paid full attention to her with what she was going to explain to us about it.

With our attention, the nurse professionally, in depth, explained to us what the things inside the bag actually were. 'They include the organs Dr Chu removed from your father in the operation,' she said, clearly pointing to it telling, which one was the part of Father's rectum with a tumour, which one was the bladder, and which one was the prostate. We looked at them, struggling to find way to breathe and failing to ask anything.

The nurse then asked us if we had any questions to consult with the doctor and, if there was any family member who would come later might want to have a look at it. We then replied to her that it would be enough and asked her to do next. The nurse said the tumour inside the rectum would be going through a thorough examination to get its state checked.

Chiefly, we could not but doubt if Father could live with so many vital organs Dr Chu had removed from him. At that moment we were with the nurse, what all we wanted to ask her was this question.

Father woke with eyes slightly opened after the anaesthetic wore off. All at once, we attended to him to see if he wanted anything. Curiously, out of all our expectations as his first words to us, he asked us what the time was. We could not but burst into a chuckle as an immediate response and then answering him with the time. Subsequently, we profusely praised him *excellent*, *heroic*, *bravo*—whatever words we could think of at that time—with our thumbs up, showing him this as his incentive. Never had Father been a self-conceited man for as long as we knew him—as usual, he appeared humble and with a lot of peacefulness, being as calm as he ever used to be.

Shortly after we had stayed with him with a little chat quietly, Father moved his fingers to denote us to leave, asking us to have lunch with a rather low voice with some hoarseness. Yeah, he was that humorous! We left as he said, leaving him under the watchful eyes of a band of professional nurses to take intensive care of him.

Indubitably, what Father, at this critical stage, needed most was intensive care that only the professional nurses at the hospital could provide him. As for us, we would go see him at the hospital in the days to come so we could share with him the pain he would have to suffer and give him the love and support he needed most as fuel.

May arrived in the afternoon, more than happy and excited to know that Father had successfully undergone the operation. She had not yet taken her lunch, anxious to come to Father and hoping to see him the soonest. When she approached him, Father was falling asleep and we were back from lunch. May smiled to Father, saying some nice words to him and touching his hands before being asking by us to take her lunch. With that, we accompanied her to go downstairs to the canteen. May took the food she ordered with appetite, while at the same time talking with us happily about Father and other subjects. Unexpectedly, we could find happiness in such a hard time. It was amazing, we thought.

May has played a rather significant role in the family. She takes care of the family as a calling, especially when the family is in a fix. We cannot but feel immensely grateful for her. What we find is she is not only a sister in name but in real existence, with fulfilment of obligations.

Surviving the operation was not only difficult but also having to be miraculous. However, surviving the recovery would only be an uphill battle without a miracle, brooking no mistakes at all in the whole process. We all fully realized this point, so we categorically promised to each other that we would fight the battle without reservation together with Father. Such was the *promise*, so invulnerable to break, that told us Father would definitely succeed in completing the whole recovery.

The second day after the operation, Father appeared tired and a little curious. He seemed to want to know how the situation he actually was in. Nagging or bothering others was never Father's style. He chose to swivel his head slowly to attempt to observe everything changing around him on his very own quietly, searching for the differences he could sense after the operation, trying to find out some answers to his questions. Although we all noticed what he did, we found ways to chat with him, with low voices saying to him with assurance that he was fine with the surgery and just needed more rest for now. In the intervening time, nurses attended to him, doing different kinds of care that made him sometimes feel good and sometimes feel bad.

Without doubt, lying in bed and totally relying on help and care is an insanely awful thing, especially when the one is at the same time badly ill and suffering from various sorts of pains and fears.

By the third day of luckily surviving the operation, Father began feeling some pains in the wounds of the surgery done despite the prescribed anaesthetic drip, and he came to realize that was what he would have to confront in the coming days. We noticed him having an urge to sit up or make his body turn, only to find himself unable to do so. Standing beside him, we failed to think of anything to do for him. There was an immediate heartbreak setting in. The only way to prevent the atmosphere from getting worse was to talk, and fortunately, Father grasped our good will and chatted with us with the topics we found.

No topic would be better than that of the coming Chinese Dragon Boat Festival that we would find it interesting and meaningful. We initiated it with the sticky rice dumplings Father and Mother make for us every year on this day. Father immediately appeared a bit more cheerful than before, talking about how he and Mother made the dumplings. He told us the whole process from buying the ingredients in markets, comparing the quality and price of them from store to store, to having them boiled in some big pots in the kitchen at home for hours and hours enduring the immense heat. At last, he told us how satisfied he and Mother were when the dumplings came out served as handsome and tasting good. Chiefly, he spoke more than we did, and we could not be happier to see him this way. We let him talk, being glad to be his listeners, with us sometimes smiling and sometimes laughing as his reward.

The Dragon Boat Festival, falling on the fifth day of the fifth lunar month every year, is a day on which all Chinese communities will be going to commemorate. It marks the memorial day of the death of a loyal official named Qu Yuan at the time of Sung Dynasty in Chinese history. The legend has that the official, after the emperor had denied all his remonstrations, sacrificed by drowning himself in the sea to show loyalty to the emperor and the dynasty. When people knew that he had drowned, they threw dumplings into the sea to feed the fish with a view of preventing them from eating his body. Although such an episode of history is sad and lamentable, the story of the dumplings was successfully made into such a legend that it was passed on from generation to generation in the Chinese communities regardless of how many people will still earnestly remember such a section of history.

'This year, you all have to buy them in markets,' Father continued. 'Don't worry next year. Next year, Mother and I will again make them for all of you.' He could not stop saying. We just laughed and laughed, offering him our best wishes and saying to him, 'Of course, next year we want more. You and Mother have to make more, for we find they are far more delicious than those sold in the markets!'

Obviously, we could tell how painful it was being ill, staying at the hospital and being unable to be with their loved ones, especially in festivals.

We all learned that Father would have quite a way to go to make recovery, and we fully understood it required not only the capability of his whole body's function but also crucially his mental tenacity. Given any octogenarian, it would only be a grim, grim challenge for him.

May called me, expressing to me some of her feelings. She said she was very much worried, saying she was afraid Father might give up—she had once or twice peeped at him revealing a face of affliction. She said she was sad seeing Father suffer. 'That's my feeling too, sister. However, try not to think of anything negative. The only way to answer such a challenge the family has never encountered is be positive.' I replied to her as a way of consolation. We two sisters, sharing a lot of love growing up together like a pair of twins, always reveal our feelings to each other without hiding. As with any such call, we could talk for over an hour.

Today, Father appeared a bit off beam after discovering that there were *two* artificial excretory openings, not one as he expected, made for his liquid and solid waste excretion respectively. They were located on the two sides of his abdomen. Before the operation, we had seen Dr Chu in his clinic, listening to him explaining the situation Father was in. He said he would remove Father's bladder when there was a necessity, and he could only judge without fail as soon as he cut open the abdomen when the operation was underway. Therefore, Father now realized that his bladder was gone in the operation with the two openings he now found. He seemed feeling a bit worried.

Back then, we threw this critical judgment onto Dr Chu, trusting him to be professional enough on one hand, and on the other hand, we had asked him to go all out to help Father preserve his bladder if possible. He then further explained to us that there would be one opening made for the solid waste excretion if the bladder would be good enough to preserve. As to the opening for solid waste excretion, it would also be temporary, with him saying there would be a second and small operation to close the opening a few weeks after the first operation was done.

Father was a person who could better accept facts than anyone can. Once he knew the bladder was gone—meaning there would forever be a opening, making him forever carry a bag for urine excretion—he said humorously to us, 'It's not bad. I don't have to spend time to pee in washroom,' with a slight chuckle. We stood beside him laughed too.

Yeah, Father's life axiom was 'When you cannot beat them, join them'. When there is no way out, find a way out. When you cannot find a way out, stay calm and try not to exaggerate. When pessimism holds swing, be all the more optimistic. He was always a person of deeds and words in chorus.

On his fourth day lying in bed, Father began to be able to move his body slowly and successfully got out of bed to a chair—of course, with an enormous help from the nurses. When I saw him this afternoon, he sat on the chair, gazing out through the broad and seemingly seamless window at the stunning view. At first, I thought he was enjoying the view, only to learn what he was thinking afterward. Whenever I did not know what he thought, I looked affectionately at him and asked him about it. 'Nothing' was, more often than not, his reply to me. Father did not lie, so I saw he really did not have anything serious to think of.

However, Father, as if opening up a topic, talked with me this time about some of his feelings about the past few days. 'Lying in bed and being unable to move even a little bit was a lot more painful than death.' He said. Truly, he was tied somewhere to the bed in the first two days right after the operation to prevent him from moving lest any move should reopen the wounds the operation had done. 'Unable to turn my body from side to side, I felt my back severely burnt,' Father recounted. 'And now I know how painful and torturing it has been being for your grandmother, long condemned to a bed for almost ten years.' He sighed. Seldom did Father mention life's pains. This time was the first time ever I heard him mention about this topic. At that very moment, I fully got him, and at the same time, my heart broke at feeling the excruciating pain he had suffered.

'Yes, Father, Grandmother is suffering, and we cannot do much for her except seeing her more.' I replied to him with both of my hands touching his. In fact, the 'Grandmother' Father mentioned is his mother-in-law. Father lived a life of respecting and loving everyone around him, extending to all relationships.

At that point, Father still could not eat despite him getting a great appetite to do so. What he said to us was that he felt very hungry every minute, not to mention every midnight. A medical tube embedding into a small blood vessel in one of his hands after the operation was to provide him nutrition. 'This tube could only mean nutrition for me but could not make my stomach full,' he said, pointing at it and showing contempt despite a smile. Oddly enough, we were happy to hear him call for food. Perhaps, we thought, when a patient resumes eagerness to eat with appetite, it should be a symbol of making progress towards the very first stage of recovery. Undoubtedly, recovery at this part was crucial and indispensable to Father, and none of us dared to take it lightly.

Dr Chu came every day, attending to Father. However, we were not there every time he came. Thus, Father would sometimes repeat to us what Dr Chu had said to him. Today, he said Dr Chu gave him a thumbs-up after pressing his abdomen to examine if the colon inside was working after the operation. He then said Dr Chu praised him as superb. "'I have never seen an old man like you able to suffer so much pain without fear or a word of blame.'" Father recounted Dr Chu as saying.

We could not help laugh and applaud. Yeah, nothing would be happier and more encouraging than hearing Father's situation was progressing. "'But, you still could not eat. You have to be a bit patient. It would likely happen in a few days, when the colon works further better.'" Father continued to quote what Dr Chu said.

Ten days rolled by after the operation. Father, had eventually passed the most critical stage of the recovery. We felt more than blessed to have this ideal result, which we had only dared to pray but did not expect before. What we would do next was our utmost to help Father in the process of recovery.

With one bag slapping on one side of his abdomen and the other hanging down beside the bed, Father knew the rest of his life would not be as easy as before to live. He had to learn how to take care of the bags in the first place, he thought. Nurses came to Father, asking him whom he lived with and suggesting such people to learn how to deal with the bags first, and then Father himself.

We all respectively were married and left the family long ago, having our own families, and this was when Mother, now and in the past ten-odd years, lived with Father. They relied heavily and solely on each other in taking care of themselves in terms of daily necessities.

Reasonably, Mother would be the first one who had this obligation to learn changing the bags Father had to carry after discharged from the hospital and going back home. Unluckily, Mother was not so willing to take on such duty. She explained to us that she believed she would be incompetent in doing this job because she could not stand the smell of that stuff. She was honest, and we wanted to see her expressing her real feelings to us without disguise so we could find solutions.

Among us siblings, Sam lived nearest to Father and Mother. He promised to undertake without reservation the job Mother seemed to be delegating upon him. Thereby, he learned how to change the bags with the nurses' tutelage. Within just three lessons he took, he said he could manage to do it and asked us not to worry. We were not only relieved a lot but also thanked him for his help. It is certain that only if you really love someone would you not fear or disgust the smell or sight of that stuff and be willing to do it. We found Sam happened to work—he had the conditions required. We could not but feel a great deal of gratefulness for him.

What Father was hospitalized in was a private hospital, one of the most expensive and renowned ones, famous in Hong Kong as being for the haves. Owing to the point that we are not that rich and Father was an uninsured, we had to pay out of pocket for the fees both of the hospital and the doctor charged. Many times, Father had wanted to thank us using his language and facial expression. Nevertheless, what we wanted him to do in return was not to thank us but do his utmost in recovery and live happily and easefully in the remaining time of his life he and we deserved.

One main reason why Father would receive cure in a private hospital was he had no choice when the doctors in the public hospitals said to us that they were not daring enough to perform so big and risky an operation to so senior and weak an old man.

Today, July 1, was the memorial day of Hong Kong's sovereignty reverting to China from Britain since 1997. It is a big day every year for most of the people in Hong Kong and China. Rationally, many would like to avail themselves of this occasion to celebrate in a variety of ways with their loved ones or friends. Simultaneously, there would also be not a few people taking to the streets staging protests against the government and appealing for different issues. It is impressive not only to this place but also to the rest of the world! Such a democratic scene that created by Hong Kong people with their unremitting efforts and endeavour done in pursuing democracy is paid off. As to us, the fireworks, a main event every year holding at night to conclude a whole day's celebration, would be our treat.

Having heard Father was able to try eating some fluid food, we jubilantly went to the hospital to check it out. For *thirteen days*, completely relying on a nutrition medical tube, Father spent the first time in his life without swallowing food for such a long time. We could not wait to see how he would look like when he ate, when what we thought of him would be more than amazing.

The big day falling on a Sunday, most of the working class were entitled to a holiday, and we too enjoyed such a privilege. With that, we all went see Father far earlier; and as a result, there were far more of us at a time in a room than usual. Seeing so many of us there with him, Father remained lying in bed, offering us sometimes a slight smile and sometimes a low-voiced conversation. In fact, we had not seen him eat thus far. We just heard the nurse say he had taken a spoon of congee in the morning.

May arrived near evening, and as soon as she got to Father, she could not stop asking him what he had for breakfast and lunch and what he would like to have the coming dinner. We four siblings whereupon took out the menu the hospital's canteen provided to have a thorough reading, suggesting this and that. We exchanging ideas, saying this would be good because we had tried it before and it tasted nice, or that would also be good because we had also tried it earlier and it did not taste bad. The room suddenly turned into a canteen with an ambiance of much appetite. Father looked at us, smiling and nodding in response to whatever we suggested him.

Clearly, we were very *happy* to find out what Father's situation actually was.

Finally, we had ordered rice noodles with pork broth for Father. When it came, Father had it placed on the small table, saying he would take it later when he wanted. A whole day entertaining guests was not that easy as a patient; Father looked tired but remained always looking at us. We knew he was tired, but we did not want to leave, however. We four siblings wanted to see him eat—especially, we wanted to serve him on his side.

Father signalled us to leave. He said, 'You all should be hungry. Go take dinner, and then enjoy the fireworks later on.' Although we had a strong eagerness to stay to see him eat, we actually knew he was tired and might want to take a real rest. Therefore, we said goodbye to him happily without further probing into the subject of his eating. We thought we should let him take his course.

Amid all the episodes during the visit today, there was one I found so touching that it almost made me cry. From morning to dusk, Father might find himself lying in bed for so long that he would sometimes want to turn or even sit up. He asked Sam to help him make it. The scene was *unforgettable*, with every step ingrained into my eyes. Sam first gently held Father's upper body up from the bed and then gently pulled his feet down from the edge of the bed. Obviously, it sapped some strength from both of them.

Father sat on one side of the bed with feet down, facing us and smiling contentedly at Sam and us. We all noticed him wanting to try another harder movement, but we did not know what it was. Shortly after sitting on the bed with feet downwards to the floor, catching his breath for minutes, we saw him indicating to Sam that he wanted to try to stand. Sam did not tell him no but attended to his wish. He made the effort as far as he could to hold him up, and when Father eventually stood after rising with a wobble, Sam immediately hugged him tightly. The scene was a big and warm hug of a father and a son, so touching that I thought I would never forget it in my life.

Other than the special emotion I had, I found the scene so touching because ever since I have had sense in my life, Father had projected to me an image of a beefy man who could never be defeated. Illness and ageing collaborated to make him turn into so weak a person that I could not witness. Inexorably, it is the revelation of life!

When we were about to finish the dinner, we called the nurses at the hospital to see if Father had taken the noodles we ordered and viewed the fireworks through the window. 'The fireworks were viewed, but the noodles remain full.' One of the nurses who frequently attended to Father replied to us with some humour.

We all knew Father would not be able to resume eating at one swoop. We thought it might have to take a little more time trying and trying. What we thought then was, all the same, positive. We conveyed to each other a message that Father's situation was normal. The ground we held was that when a person stops eating for a rather long period, his stomach must have some effects, and when such a person resumes taking food—even the most fluid food—his stomach has to take time to adapt. It should be no point to rush, when such a situation admits of great latitude.

The next day, nurses told us that Father vomited the previous midnight.

Undaunted by any bad news, what we did at that moment was looked forward with optimism. We only allowed ourselves to think this way—that was when Father could not eat today, so he might be able to eat tomorrow. When tomorrow he still could not eat, he would be able to eat the day after tomorrow, and so forth. Such belief was so strong that we would see any news as just news.

Although Father had to stop trying taking food today, he did not appear bad. He talked with us like the past ten odd days he did. As to us, we did not talk about eating lest he should have a feeling that we urged him to eat. When we tried to find some other subjects to talk about with him, Father opened up the subject of eating to us without worries. "'You could eat now. Why not get some food to eat?'" Father cited what Dr Chu said to him this morning. He then said to us that he replied to the doctor naughtily with a shrug that he just did not want to eat for now but later.

The story went that after the operation, Father could not stop asking Dr Chu when he could eat every time he attended to him, and every time, his reply to Father was it would be soon and he should be patient. When he was so eager to take some food, Father found Dr Chu's reply to him lacked compassion. It turned out a bit ironic that when Dr Chu found he could start eating yesterday, he was failing to do so. Therefore, he tried to play a trick onto Dr Chu when he found the doctor intentionally asking him about eating this morning. Father deliberately made some humour on the reply to him.

Today, third of July, Father finally could try a small bowl of rice with fish. When I arrived, he was taking it. I thought I was lucky enough to have had seen that. He ate and ate, describing how tasty the fish was, and I looked and looked at him, feeling so happy finding out he eventually could eat. It was his lunch— the first lunch he had while staying at the hospital. He had rice and fish after starving for half a month. Although he could eat, he still needed the nutrition tube to help maintain a stable and normal life. That meant Father still had quite a long way to go, although with everything that Father was now giving us, we had great confidence in his recovery.

Owing to the blood vessel, the medical nutrition tube embedding for quite a long time in his hand appeared overburdened, turning into a kind of black colour. Today, Father needed to do a transplant—to remove the tube and embedding it into another blood vessel in another hand. The process was smooth, and Father seemed to feel nothing. Did it not cause pain? We doubted that!

Father used to hide the pain in front of us to avoid us growing sad.

After either lying in bed or sitting on a chair for more than half a month, Father had a great eagerness trying to walk. With the approval of the nurses, Father asked Sam and Mother to help him about it. The result was, the two flanked him on both sides as he walked, holding his hands and arms tightly along with the medical nutrition tube rack. The scene of the three walking was exceptionally warm and sentimental. Father smiled, looking like an infant learning to walk with curiosity, with his eyes checking if anything could impress him on the way. Sam and Mother paid full attention and strength to offer aid, brooking no mistakes on each step they all took. Although Father walked so slowly that it took almost a minute to finish just a step, it was already more than amazing. As fragile as he was, he insisted on walking more steps with no regard to what we asked him to take five. We could feel that Father was happy to find him able to walk. It has adequately afforded us a lesson, teaching us that life is eventually beautiful if only you know how to experience it with appreciation. Every experience—good or bad, easy or difficult—is worth us not only undergoing but also appreciating.

Shortly after taking less than ten steps, Father could not but stop. As we could see, he was more than tired. He signalled Sam it was enough. Sam not only got him but also realized that he could not walk back to his bed. He then asked the nurses to provide

Father a wheelchair. In a minute, Father was on the wheelchair, aided by a nurse, and was back into his room. Sam helped the nurse in making Father comfortable on the bed. Mother and we looked at them all that time, preparing ourselves at any moment to provide help also. We all smiled, seeing the walk as the vital first successful step of recovery.

Step by step—there would eventually be a step closest to the full recovery one day.

The next day, Father again was eager to walk with the good memory of the previous day's first-time walking experience after the operation. He repeated the series of procedures with Sam and Mother the previous day they did, and took the steps with more courage and confidence than he had yesterday. It turned out he walked clearly a bit faster than yesterday, along with some smiles he wore on his face from time to time that could not hide. Sam could not but feel proud with such a strong-willed man beside him as his father. At the same time, he made a joke to the nurses watching them, saying, 'Beware of him. He can walk now. He may sneak out!' All the nurses burst into laughter in such a moving scene all of a sudden.

Life will be something when we spend it in a positive way— this was our newest motto.

The recovery seemed to have a good start, we all thought. Seeing how Father did not utter even a word of gripe or blame during the very first stage after the operation despite suffering an immense pain, and seeing how he smoothly came to this stage eating and walking, we were on the assumption that the recovery would definitely be a reality.

Amazingly, Father began asking when he could go home. What an inspiring question! Inspiring question though it was, Dr Chu found it a bit aggressive and he wanted Father to stay at the hospital a bit longer. Without doubt, it was a literal fact that so old a man having undergone so big an operation should be taken care a lot more carefully than the younger ones, and more importantly, we all realized that things would relentlessly turn bad once anything went wrong at home. As we knew only hospital could provide him such intensive and professional care he needed most. Father accepted what Dr Chu had advised him, nodding and smiling, saying it was not bad to be staying there with so many people taking care of him. 'It is so relaxing being at loose end.' Father said with humour.

CHAPTER TWO

It was not easy to have Father come this far when he was able to go back home after staying for twenty-six days at the hospital, completing the very first and critical stage of the recovery with the help of a march of professional nurses. We all were proud of the success. Before waving them goodbye, we exchanged comfort and nice words with the nurses who had always attended to Father. Undeniably, the scene a patient coming out of the hospital happily is the most *beautiful* picture in the world. We deeply felt grateful and blessed for what had appeared in front of our eyes.

We clapped and laughed while taking Father home with the van we arranged in advance. We could not be happier to see Father smile so lively to us, and we could tell by his smiles that he was very much appreciative for what we had done for him. Father, what we felt, you know, was having you suffer so much pain to keep alive staying with us, and we thought we should be ten times more appreciative than you were. We indeed felt very, very much thankful to you!

Profusely asking Mother for food, Father seemed to turn into a famine refugee after he was back from the hospital. Nevertheless, we all saw it a sign of auspiciousness, a good-luck token of a patient making recovery. Apart from suddenly believing in superstition, we all the time have held a strong belief in science and chose to think tilting towards this direction. As a person after an operation without genuinely taking food for a long time, he ought to be hungry. It was more than normal. Therefore, Mother tried to cook what Father wanted to eat every meal to satisfy not only his appetite but also mainly his seemingly ever-empty stomach.

Mother would sometimes notify us of Father's situation. Among what she said, what we heard most was that he ate a lot, along with some practices he did every day: he walked to a park, he bought some casual stuff like newspaper, he watched television on the sofa with snacks, and awesomely, he did some simple light housework. That was, he almost could do everything as before. What was happening now was *fabulous*, we thought.

Today, a Sunday, we went home to play mah-jong with Father for the first time when he was coming back home from the hospital.

Father had so few hobbies that what we could play with him was mah-jong most of the time.

Mah-jong is a game involving four persons that has fair and interesting rules to follow. Just learning the rules is entertaining enough. A complete game includes east, south, west, and north rounds, with each having at least four games. After finishing a full round, it will be started again from east to north.

Everyone is on a level playing field over the mah-jong table. The enchantment of the game lies not only on wins or losses but also lies on its weird and unique features you will every time find shrouded in mysteries that you can never understand or find out. While one game can bring out your best in luck, another can easily bring out your worst in character. While one game can inspire you, another can frustrate you. As to the performance, it depends on the way and the skill of all the involved people who play, but not only yours. To the zenith, one can affect another's fate with his or her unique skill to play with different luck. Regarding us, we usually played it as a communication or leisure in most of the gatherings. Still, we found mah-jong incredibly awesome!

After getting some noodles Mother prepared for us, we went to the mah-jong table to have a showdown with each other. As it was the first time to play this game with Father after he had undergone an operation, there was the following question raised: could Father play it as well as before? We had no idea. We four siblings had secretly discussed about it earlier this morning behind Father, and it would be soon for us to find out.

When the game started, Father acted as he used to be, calm and silent. We too acted as what we used to act, we chatted, and we played. As we played, we at the same time discharged of our duty to observe every motion of Father, including his facial expressions. The observation we had was that every movement Father made was a lot slower than it was in the past. Nevertheless, we thought it normal when we found him wearing a slight smile on his face all the time and enjoying playing the game with us along with sometimes uttering a sound or having a short conversation. We were sure that he was good and complacent.

After completing playing a full circle—east, south, west, and north—we asked Father if he needed taking a break. 'No, just go on.' He replied to us firmly. Yeah, Father's words were always short and expressive. 'Good,' we then replied to him, with our voices a bit higher to support him in return. The game played on.

Another full circle completed, Father finally felt tired, but he appeared happily. He took the initiative, saying to us that he needed a rest before us demanding. We laughed and accompanied him to his bed. When he was lying down properly on the bed with one thick layer of blanket covering him from neck to feet despite the sweltering weather, we four siblings went on the mah-jong game. When Father made a lot of endeavour in his recovery after surgery hoping to restore his health to normal by staying with us, we dared not take anything lightly in taking care of him to upset any effort he made. It might be that, in a way, we looked like we were taking care of a child sometimes.

Playing was the only way when Father took a rest. We four siblings essentially chatted over the mah-jong table instead of focusing on the game, mainly revealing to each other face to face, without hiding, the happy feeling mixed with some unspeakable sentiments in seeing Father this way after we had been all-out fighting the battle with him.

The role love plays in life is so overwhelming that it is peremptory. It is certainly true that love can make miracles.

Deep down, we knew how strong Father was to have had come this far since he had been ill. To all intents and purposes, Father suffered from the ailment long, long ago, probably two to three years ago. The reason he had not sought cures was that he concealed the illness from us, explaining later to us that he did not want us to worry. He alone suffered on one side, and on the other, he let Sam bring him to see a practitioner for another kind of remedy—herbal cure. What Father did could be unwise, but his kindness in doing it was self-evident. Such was the kindness he bestowed upon us that made us love him more.

More than clearly, the practitioner who cured Father was far from competent, causing Father's illness to deteriorate going from bad to worse. Without earnestly diagnosing what Father had developed, the practitioner prescribed him herbs every time, saying it would heal the problems Father had and charging expensive costs. Not until days before the last Father's Day, when Father was hanging by a thread and lying in bed after being rushed to hospital did the whole story get told.

Based on the story told, there had been almost two to three years in that intervening time when Father first found himself uncomfortable. Therefore, we fully understood how much Father had suffered alone physically and mentally while concealing his situation from us. The fault could be with all of us. Even if it was not a fault, it was our carelessness. We should have concerned about his health more by frequently asking after him. For now, realizing that crying over spilt milk would only be a wild goose chase, what we were going to do was to get Father the best cure and care to make recovery and live happily.

One thing we profoundly grasped was that Father chose to hide the truth from us as a way of showing his love. He did not want us to worry or fear, and we had no words to thank him in this light.

Although Father said he needed a rest, he actually did not sleep. He chose to hear our voices, our laughter, and the sound of mah-jong. He woke far earlier than we expected, watching us play and finding food to eat. At the very present, no scene in front of our eyes could be lovelier than the scene of Father looking for food to eat. Father, you were so lovely! What you had showed us was that we should be happy and grateful for everything we have, and we should never try to desperate look for the things that are beyond our reach to bring about sadness and unhappiness. You were far more amazing than we have all along thought of you, and such amazement was really something pretty special inside you that you had never shown us or we had never been caring enough to find out. Were we too late to discover this—yes, we were—so it was time we had to catch up.

At dinner, Father appeared unusually happy with eyes *shining*. A bowl of rice, a little meat, a little vegetable, a little beans, and finally a little beer—despite all being little amounts, Father saw them as *big* enough to be a feast. Father ate them with as much pleasure and gratefulness as he used to have for any meal before. As for us, we chatted with each other, talking about how tasty the food was, comparing this with that, drinking beer with Father, and wishing him good health. Such a dinner was really a godsend, we thought. We did not know whom we had to say thanks to, so we thanked every god we could name in chorus by toasting together.

Seeing Father having no problem in taking care of himself with some help of Sam and Mother, we felt not only relieved but also proud.

Every time when we looked back, we would invariably appear a mixture of feeling. At the time when we knew Father was terribly ill, John, against the clock, searched for information over the Internet about the ailment Father unluckily got, aiming at finding him the most prestigious doctor with the most effective remedial cure. That time was the most urgent moment ever in our lives, brooking no delay in catching every minute lest we should fail to survive the consequence of any procrastination.

Fortunately, John could finally find Father the doctor who was not only prestigious but also daring, courageous enough to run a big and risky operation on an octogenarian without hesitation. We, without doubt, vouched for his confidence, throwing Father's life in his hands without reserve.

Before the operation about to come, John explained to us what he had searched via the Internet, saying he was not too worried about the success of the operation but the success of the recovery. According to the information provided on the Internet, John said, not many could survive the recovery due to the scale of the devastation of the body done by the operation—especially when it was happening to someone elderly. John said we could only pray for the most desired result but in no way see it as guaranteed.

This conclusion was due to Father's situation being almost the worst, with the tumour developed in the colon growing so absurdly big. It had already pressed or even implanted partly into the bladder, leaving the bladder one-third of its original volume to store urine. This, turning out, made Father not only need to pee awful frequently every day and night, but also even hardly sat down in the latter stage. Dr Chu warned that if he did not get the operation in the soonest, the illness would threaten his life anytime. In this case, we had no alternative but one—having

Father undergo the operation, which was the riskiest. After that, what we could do was to look forward positively with optimism and do our utmost.

Luckily, Father was unexpectedly brave too, by having us decide the operation for him without choice. 'You decide' was always his words to us. Of course, we had explained to him, through and through, the health problems occurring to his body with the illness posed on him. At last, how the operation would restore his health to normal and good.

After staying at home making a recovery for twenty days, Father knew the second operation would draw near. It would be a rather *nice* operation. However nice, it was still ultimately an operation—none of us dared to take it lightly. Recently, we even discussed behind Father about it when we gathered, arguing if it was an operation Father must take.

Dr Chu had explained the above said operation to us as early as the first time we brought Father to his clinic. The upcoming operation would be rather small, especially when compared with the previous one Father had, and the aim of it was to close one of the artificial excretory openings currently located on Father's abdomen (for solid waste excretion), letting Father only need to carry one bag in the future (for excretion of urine). It sounded more convenient and comfortable for Father's life afterwards if the operation would come to fruition. The method was to cut open a small hole over his abdomen to have the edge of two parts of the inside colon cut apart before being attached again.

As sound as it would be, we prayed for every possible blessing to Father, hoping he would undergo it without a hitch. Appointment made, for the second time, Father went to the hospital, bracing for the second operation he would deal with. This time; however, he had a lot more of light-heartedness than the previous one he had.

It was early August, a rather hot day. We accompanied Father in heading to the hospital he stayed last time. Before checking in, we had a lunch with him, letting him eat whatever he wanted to eat at a restaurant. Wonderfully, he ate exceptionally well, showing no sign of fear of the operation, but a sign of optimism he especially had this time.

Father seemed very much familiar with the procedures of the stay at the hospital. He knew far better than any one of us what he would be doing. Once settling down, a series of procedures started. Checks on this and that within his body done by the nurses and recorded as references as a prelude. In the meantime, Father would take rests or watch TV programs with the computer the hospital provided which hung from the ceiling above his bed. After staying for twenty-six days last time in the same hospital, Father managed to deal with everything around him without us worrying.

Morning came. We all arrived on time before Father was into the surgery room. Father waved us good morning, and we blew him our kisses. The atmosphere this time was obviously far better than the last time. Even the nurses appeared light-hearted, greeting us with smiles. Finally, Father was sitting on a wheelchair heading to the surgery room. We supported him with loud voices, saying we would see him later. Father again smiled and nodded, appearing as peaceful and calm as he used to be. Father, you were awesome!

We heard Dr Chu say the operation would take around an hour, so we went downstairs, having our breakfast and chat. Time sneaks in usual days but stays in unusual days. During that single hour, we found it hard to pass the time and used a variety of ways to look at the watches we wore by peeping, staring, glancing, and then pretending not to worry a bit and saying to each other that it would be quick. Obviously, we could not wait to see Father coming out. Last time was a miracle—would it be again this time? There was no telling! Would luck again shower on him? There was no telling either. So many questions without answers suddenly seemed to haunt us, causing us to become a bit anxious.

Such kind of emotion might stem from the memories we got by experiencing not a little sadness and happiness with Father in the past two months, and they were still fresh in memories. Furthermore, we had literally witnessed how hard Father had done everything more than he could to overcome all the difficulties he had to face in the recovery. If the operation failed this time, it would not only ruthlessly upset all the efforts he had made before but also stood a possibility of leading him fatally. If it really happened, it would be the worst chapter in our lives. We dared not think of such scene. After all, we chose to think positively that Father should deserve far better, with his extraordinary strong will and effort, a longer life with happiness. We then, from time to time, prayed for god's mercy to again shower on him.

Sam's mobile rang, and he could not wait to pick it up. Happily, the call was from a nurse who informed us that Father was back in his room, waiting for us. We rushed upstairs at once with joy and laughter to get to Father.

Father lay in bed, appearing more than conscious except that he was moaning the pain from the wound he felt intolerable. He seemed unable to take that pain, showing us a rather pained face such that we could not but ask for the nurses. The nurse attending to Father explained that the dose of the anaesthetic prescribed might not have been enough to ease the pain the wound caused. She subsequently increased the dose of it to see if it could make Father feel better. Once the increment was added, Father was immediately relieved not a little, starting to talk with us about his feeling.

We stood by him smiling, praising his bravery, asking him how he felt, and saying to him that he would be better and better henceforward with only one bag needed to carry after this operation. He smiled back to us with eyes sometimes open and sometimes half-closed replying to us, 'Yes, sure.' Clearly, he was happy despite being tired and desperate to take a rest. We too got a bit tired, sat for a while beside him, and then left.

Dr Chu said Father only had to take about a week hospitalized, adding he had never seen so old a patient with such a strong will. He asked us to take care of Father when he got back home.

The day after the operation, Father's first question to Dr Chu was 'When can I eat?' This time Dr Chu answered him with more light-heartedness, saying, 'It would be quick, it would be quick.'

Today when we went see him, Father already could appear well enough to talk to us with smiles and humour. He seemed to have a beautiful picture conjured up on his mind depicting how the rest of his life would go on, and he showed us a big unstoppable smile. To our knowledge, what Father had all along expected his life to be was not the luxurious one but a humble one. Father used to live his life in the simplest and the most uncomplicated way. Besides, Father had the extraordinary attribute of being able to confront life's hardships more than anyone we have known; we could not but admire him.

The third day after the operation, Father finally could eat. After passing some check-up over his abdomen by Dr Chu, Father could try to eat some soft food. Mother brought him some congee with meat and fish, and Father gulped it down all into his stomach like a long-starving refugee. We all teased him on the surface, but we were very much delighted underneath.

Day by day, a week flew. Father was discharged from the hospital for the second time, happily going back home. Coincidently, it was his Chinese lunar birthday. Thereby, we got an idea going to a restaurant to have a small celebration first before going home. Food now became the apple of Father's eye, we joked. We began to be jealous of the food Father coveted, and we found we four siblings became the second best of his. Nevertheless, we were more than delighted about it deep down. We ordered a table of food ranging from Chinese dim sum as the main course and a few plates of noodles as secondary. We tried as far as letting Father eat whatever his appetite allowed him to take, and wonderfully, he ate far better than we thought.

We observed the way Father ate, smacking of much meticulousness. He first got a little of every variety of the food we ordered, like a gourmet tasting food. When the food went into his mouth, he chewed and chewed, and 'Good' was the word frequently coming out from him in return. We sat one next to the other to form a circle, chatting, eating, and mainly looking at Father to see if he could eat well. We just thought of how wonderful our Father was, and such was the wonderfulness that told us life was worth living no matter what. Yeah, from the time when Father got badly sick to the time he went through the cure, suffering immense pain, he had not uttered a word of blame or gripe. Furthermore, to prevent us from seeing him suffer pains and growing sad, he adopted a way of keeping silent and calm when the pain reigned him in ruthlessly and going all out in swallowing every bit of it on his own.

You were more than great, Father! We love you, and we have to learn from you about life. What we see from you is that sadness can by no means forever reign over a life but will eventually give way to happiness. Only if you do not blame anyone on your way will life be different. The laws of life are thus, and thus is life dictated so.

Driven back home in the van we arranged for earlier, Father appeared a little more talkative than usual, saying at one time how boring it was staying at the hospital and at another depicting how nice and caring the nurses there were to take care of him. 'In short, no place like home.' He suddenly said in a rather high voice. We all shared his sentiment, commending him as being smart to have such a conception about home. Laughter abounded the van, as if it was like a dose of salts, we reached home oblivious of how long the van ride had taken. Yeah, life is a thief stealing our time clandestinely when we are spending it happily.

Perceivably, everybody has a feeling that life always sneaks in at the time of happiness. This can explain the reason why we will invariably cling to happy moments like hell and store these in the best part of our memories as *treasure*.

The first thing Father did upon reaching home was walked around the house like a detective searching. He missed the house so much, we thought. Shortly, he sat at the table, asking Mother for food. We thought he might have forgotten he had just taken not a little food at the restaurant. We laughed and laughed, reminding him of the food he ate earlier. 'So snacks! I want snacks!' He smiled back at us while saying this. Going on with recovery was now Father's aim, and we could not wait for the moment to see him completely recovered and to celebrate.

Mother would sometimes report Father's situation to us. Most of the time, she mentioned how he ate.

Mother can be a caring person in a way, only that she was born with kind of a hot temper. Younger than Father by eleven years, though, she grows old with not a few health problems occurring to her these past few years—mainly heart disease posed on her recently that made her a lot physically weaker than the past. Despite all that, the two lived with and heavily relied on each other for almost sixteen years when Sam and John both were married and moved away. Conceivably, things would be very different when time rolled by sixteen years, not to mention when it was happening to the seniors.

Over the past twenty-odd years, we gradually married and moved and had our own families and children. When our kids their grandchildren were small, Father and Mother played with them as a blessing and enjoyment. The house could easily fill with sound and laughter, and their hearts could easily fill with love and warmth when the children were playing with them. Now, the children were growing up, each having their own world and getting less and less of a motivation to be with them, leaving their grandfather and grandmother's hearts not a few vacancies that *nothing* can fill.

However, Father used to appear a lot more yielding than Mother is in terms of the situation changing. Seldom did we hear him complain about things as Mother always does. Presumably, such striking difference between the two could make them supplementary to each other. Nevertheless, it could not prove to be the case all the time. Mother used to nag at people including to her most loved ones. She could easily talk Father's ear off sometimes, even for nothing. Father, a real man, used to let her talk, blaming or scolding on condition that it was tolerable enough to prevent things from getting worse. Thanks, Father, you are great. We have to thank for you kindness in this respect.

What Father ate each morning were two big-sized boiled eggs and some bread. It is common sense that recovery requires a lot of nutritious food to help progressing in the process. Mother grasped it as well and understood that at this critical moment, Father needed good food with a lot of protein, so she tried her best to provide him food leaning towards this trend.

Father, in return, ate the food Mother made with a lot of appetite. As for lunch and dinner, he would sometimes say what food he wanted to eat and ask Mother to make it for him. Most of the time, he would eat what Mother cooked. When Mother complained about how tired she was making this and that to cater to Father, we would laugh and make jokes behind her back, saying she was like a servant to Father at present when Father was hers in the past.

Father continued to make inroads in his recovery. He endeavoured by wisely being patient and keeping a happy mood. On the surface of him, everything seemed going all right. On the inside, it did not seem to be as well. He had to make solid waste excretions more than *ten times* every day after the last operation, with the artificial excretory opening over his abdomen closed. Although we knew the whole recovery would easily take half a year for an old man, including the appearance of frequent and irregular excretion, we still worried about it. We could not know if it would be an anomaly, or if we were just too much in a hurry about the completion of the recovery.

Today, Father had an appointment with Dr Chu in his clinic to have a body check-up for the first time of the follow-up consultation after undergoing operation twice. We all appeared excited despite being a bit nervous, not knowing if the result would come out proving good. Father, as usual, appeared calm and silent, having Chinese tea with us in a nearby restaurant as a warm-up. He smiled when he ate, looking like he was not a bit worried about the coming check-up. Yes, that was our Father – silent, strong as well as calm.

Dr Chu greeted us with hello before offering Father his solicitudes. Shortly after asking Father some casual questions, he did some other intensive check-ups that required both of them to go to another room, and we waited outside and chatted quietly.

After about twenty minutes, they came out, both wearing smiles. Dr Chu told us that Father's recovery was progressing satisfactorily, and more inspiring, all the scans that examined the inner parts of his abdomen proved good; if the result of the blood test coming out in a few days could prove the rate of cancer low, we could hail it an initial success of recovery. Even so, we could not help laughing and holding Father in our arms, offering him our nicest words with happy tears in our eyes. Yeah, the hardest time was out. There was no time like the present.

Father said a little, preferring to let us talk and being our loyal listener. We first talked about how strong Father's will was, praising him as courageous enough to take the operation that involved huge risks especially given no guarantee both to his survival of the operation and his recovery. Then we talked about how smart John was to find Father the most daring and competent doctor. We talked about how progressive and sophisticated today's medicine was to cure even some kinds of deadly maladies, leading many of us to a longer life expectancy. We talked about how merciful God was to spare Father a life twice in the operation room. We talked about how powerful our love was to make us come together to fight the battle with Father and to conjure up one miracle after another. We talked about how precious and unforgettable the experience we had undergone was and that it would definitely make us grow in strength. At last, we four siblings thanked each other and thanked Mother. Again, the van we rented abounded with voices like last time, and before we could finish all the conversations, it stopped and we reached home.

'Being at home was the most pleasant thing.' Father said. We all could not agree more. We were more than assured that everything was going forward on a right track in Father's recovery after coming back from Dr Chu's clinic and passing through a thorough body check-up. We were indeed relieved not a little. The coming days for Father would be brighter and brighter, and his life would only be better and better lived, we thought.

After surviving a big operation and then a small one lately, Father could now finally live with ease and happiness. We embraced hopes of Father living the longest and happiest. He deserved it or even more of it, we insisted.

Due to the rather old age of Father, Dr Chu, as early as the first operation started, suggested not to do any other kinds of treatment against the cancer as a follow up, like electrotherapy or chemotherapy. He said Father might not stand these kinds of treatment with so weak his body and so old his age. He added that doing so would only cause Father's body to weaken, and such a weakness might hugely decelerate the quality of his life or even carry him off.

We totally understood Dr Chu's analytical advice and took it. No matter how quick the cancer would come back, we would make Father live happily each day before it came. As to the coming days, we would pray every day for god's mercy showering on Father on one side, while on the other, we would do our best in the care Father needed. We insisted that such care admitted of no mistakes and carelessness lest any of those should be fatal to Father.

To all intents and purposes, Father did not know what exactly his situation was, for we had not explained to him every word what Dr Chu said to us. We just thought letting Father live in fear every day would only get him nowhere, what he needed most was a happy mood to think optimistically and act positively. Therefore, we said to Father that he would restore to good health if only he could recover completely, and the way to reach it was to eat well, sleep well, and play well. In return, Father grasped it all, saying to us that he knew and understood, asking us not to worry too much about him.

Few days passed by. The result of the blood test Father had undergone came out. A nurse from Dr Chu's clinic made a call to us, informing us of a piece of very good news. She said the result of the rate of cancer with Father was showing as low as that of a normal person. How uplifting it was!

CHAPTER THREE

Time flew without a trace, and it had already been a month and a half since Father finished taking the second small operation. He looked well, and everything seemed going all right with him except that he still needed to excrete more than ten times every day. However, Father had not complained about it. He instead grinned and bore it, and patiently waited for a day the times of such excretion would decrease. Yeah, Father was just that patient. That was, he could bear and endure anything more than anyone can.

Mid-Autumn Festival, one of the most harmonious and welcome Chinese festivals, can easily fill the streets at night with adults and children, who would carry their lovable lanterns of various styles and sizes while walking side by side. People would jubilantly form processions, chatting either quietly or noisily while admiring the full moon that dominates the sky with the most brilliant light. The festival chronicles an episode of a piece of Chinese history: the overthrow of the Mongols at the end of the Yuan Dynasty in the fourteen[th] century. Such a festival celebrated on the fifteen[th] day of the eighth lunar month every year afterwards is popular in all the Chinese communities. Usually, the people will share among them, especially their loved ones, moon cakes they buy or receive as the night reaches its climax, full of laughter and joy. Regarding the moon cakes, many still take delight in the traditional ones with salted duck yolk in their core symbolizing the full moon despite many new-fangled versions, including some weird ones of ice cream inside that are hard to explain to be a moon cake; however, they are scrambling the market and costing expensively.

Given that every year we would have a gathering to spend this popular festival together, there was no reason we would not do it this year. As it drew near, we had come up with an idea that we would take Father out at night for a dinner at a restaurant to have a celebration with us. Father could not help saying 'How nice it is, how nice it is!' upon hearing us suggesting it. We immediately looked at the calendar to nail down a date, calling the manager whose restaurant we used to have gatherings in to reserve us a room like before. The reservation confirmed, and we all looked forward to it with not a little euphoria.

A week quickly passed by. The day came. Father looked smart today, having breakfast as usual and then gearing himself up by having a haircut and a bath. In fact, it was still early to head for the restaurant. We found Father a little nervous, but we thought it normal. Having stayed for quite a long time at the hospital and then at home, today was his *first* time going out at night to attend a several-hour function (including mah-jong playing and dinner). In addition to some wonderful scenes, he might have some other unpleasant ones on his mind that made him worry, as he was unable to go through the function at the dinner with his weak body. Anyway, on one side, we encouraged him to do it; and on the other, we told him that whenever he got tired, we could go back home anytime. We thought, if Father could make it this time, he would restore himself not a little confidence, and he would be more and more confident henceforward in doing next and next and next . . .

Undoubtedly, everything needs a start. A good start means half a success, and finally, success breeds success.

After looking for a nice shirt that was comfortable enough to not only wear but that also naturally cover the bag on one side of his abdomen for urine excretion, Father looked for a pair of trousers. All the decent trousers for going out that were loaded inside his closet were too big for him now. Father caught napping appearing a bit rush, calling Mother for help. Luckily, Mother had already taken out one from the closet the previous night to make some draw in about the waist to fit Father's now shrinking body. After pulling up it, Father could not help saying 'Nice!' Under any circumstance, Mother would not allow Father to make a fool of himself and leading her to lose face. Mother is a very serious person with little fun.

The van we rented in advance arrived, and we all got downstairs to get in it, heading to the restaurant that we made reservations at a week ago. In the van, Father smiled and kept silent. Not wanting to give Father unnecessary pressure, we chatted as usual to make everything happening now exactly like the past gatherings we had, to make Father feel more at ease.

Within an hour, we arrived at the restaurant. We accompanied Father, walking slowly into it with much laughter and joy despite us finding he could only walk at a snail pace, carrying his still fragile body. Settling down, with everyone each getting a favourite drink, we began to play mah-jong as a warm-up before the upcoming feast with delicacies and wines.

Father sat on the chair with the position he wanted and waited to play his favourite hobby. He used to play mah-jong with us as a means of communication. Indeed, he could play it with enjoyment any time regardless of win or loss. Magically, mah-jong is a game that can bring out one's full character, not allowing one to hide even a little but expose all. Many even say mah-jong reflects a real-life drama from time to time, displaying some patterns of a life's journey.

While one game of mah-jong can be easily and smoothly done, another can, beyond all reason, brim with difficulties to such an extent that it even does not allow you to breathe when you are actually being the same person with the same skill. A game of mah-jong can upset you with twists and turns while another can delight you with unexpected ease like magic.

Mah-jong can not only see through one's weakness in disposition but also brutally bring it out in full view of the public. Simultaneously, it can stretch one's endurance in confronting difficulties and bring about their lofty in temperament as a climax. In short, mah-jong is not merely a game or gamble, it is all the more an artistic form of presenting life in its unique way.

When you are intoxicated in playing this game, it will fill you with great enchantment. Such enchantment is not just talking about win or loss but the rich axiom in it mirroring not a few patterns of our lives. A round of mah-jong can easily display before our very eyes a full life's journey, which is inevitably dotted with simplicities and difficulties. Finally, you will find only those who know the way to survive the difficulties can go through every game with real pleasure.

Nevertheless, Mah-jong is eventually a gamble; with stakes, you can make it big or small. If you play it big, the consequence is at your own risk since it will, any time, mean your life. If you play it small, you will find it not only entertaining but also educational.

Our family, only gathering for this game, used to play it as an entertainment with the smallest stakes.

Father, a person with much patience and endurance in confronting or suffering difficulties and pains, always sat on a chair with many a slight smile every time he played this game with us. Today, he played it with much more delight than before, although every step and move he took was obviously a lot slower. As slow as he was, he played it well, more than smart and clever to organize every game to attempt to win. It told his brain was much more overwhelming than his body. He employed skill to make every game the best he could, and no matter how it was easy or hard, he just kept silent. Never did he utter a word of dissatisfaction when the game appeared hard, nor would he lose temper under any circumstances.

As a game of four persons with each possessing a different personality, it is inevitable that some unpleasant scenes would sometimes occur in the process. When voices of vehement anger exploded from someone in the game, the other three may have to try their best to understand and tolerate, especially when the involved are a family. Father used to exemplify himself to us all the time in terms of such tolerance and understanding, and we, in return, usually followed his lead. Father adopted a way of grinning and bearing every hard time he faced, and we owed it to his lofty inherent integrity.

When a full round of game including east, south, west, and north finished, we asked Father if he needed to take five and got from him an answer replying nay. With so inspiring an answer, we, from the word go, could not wait to play another round with applause.

We observed that Father was really in a desirable progress about recovery, even a bit more than expected. We could not but smile and smile when we four siblings sometimes looked at each other reading it. Truly, we four knew each other so well that we could even read each other's mind. At last, Father has won the game, but not much. With a smile, he said to us, 'I'm just a bit tired but very happy.'

With that, we proceeded to the table of the dinner we had ordered. Sam and John cracked open some wine bottles, asking the waiter serving us to take out some glasses or goblets for the wine. May and I arranged the seats for the younger ones to sit on. The sound of laughter and chats crazily abounded the room, and with the help of several waiters offering us each one set of tableware, the dinner started with euphoria.

It was the first time Father had a dinner at night outside at a restaurant since he was terribly ill and afterwards staying at the hospital for cure. Given that, the first thing we did was to toast with him, wishing him good health. 'Father, good heath!' we said *at the top of our lungs* to show him our stirring sentiments. Father, in response to our zealousness, held up a glass of tea saying 'Good, good,' and drank. Yeah, we were that simple. Curiously, simple things can make us happy. The simpler we are, the happier— another new motto after coming together to battle the illness with Father. For now, no scene in the world could be more beautiful than the scene where Father smiled and felt good.

Father appeared to be hungrily gazing at every plate of the cuisine that came, stretching out his hands with sometimes chopsticks or sometimes a spoon to grab whatever he wanted to eat with some help of Sam sitting beside him. Every time the food entered his mouth, he relished the texture and the taste of it by nibbling it slowly and describing in detail. 'Nice, good taste! I want a little more . . . Enough! I want some of that,' frequently came from Father tonight. Certainly true, it was surprisingly amazing.

Carrying one bag for urine excretion slapping on one side of his abdomen seemed not to pose a problem on him, Father had already mastered the skill of changing a full bag with a new one. Nevertheless, Mother said to us that he still needed to make solid waste excretion many times a day. When we were in doubt the phenomenon normal, we did worry about it. But the last check-up did tell us that Father was progressing satisfactorily in recovery, and most importantly, the blood test came out proving his rate of cancer low. It was just few weeks ago, so we chose to think the phenomenon was normal and we waited.

The next check-up would be in the coming late November, and today was the last day of September, there were about two months in between for us to further observe how Father would progress. We concluded that at this moment, seeing him with everything being all right, we should stay with him eating and playing rather than talk about his excretion in question.

The dinner lasted about three hours, with not only delicacies but also nice conversations, before we rounded it off with everyone clinking glasses with each other, saying 'Happy Mid-Autumn Festival!' Yeah, tonight was wonderful! Every face revealed a lot of laughter and joy. Father thanked us with smiles and nods when we asked him if he had enough. A whole day's function had in effect made him a bit exhausted, but he denied it. We observed that he was very much likely to linger on such an ambiance when leaving. We understood, and we promised him there would be next and next and next in the future. We accompanied him in leaving the restaurant, and we got into the van we had arranged, heading back home.

Father's confidence was back and would become increasingly stronger with such an outdoor event smoothly and happily run, we thought.

In the van, Father seemed to fall asleep. We kept quiet to let him sleep. Within an hour, we arrived home. Father said, 'What a nice day, what a nice day,' going to his bedroom after saying goodnight to us. As we have known long, he was that simple and straightforward, a man without any unwelcome or bad disguise.

The next morning, Father woke up early, resuming the day's routine by firstly walking slowly in the garden nearby to breathe some fresh air and then buying a newspaper before returning home. At home, he used to watch television, concentrating on some programs he liked. Occasionally, he would help Mother doing some light housework. As to food, every day, he had three meals prepared by Mother and Sam carefully. In the morning, he had two boiled eggs and some bread and water. Lunch was some noodles with pork and some cabbage and then a little Chinese tea. Dinner was a bowl of rice with different kinds of food such as fish, pork, chicken, and sometimes duck, and vegetables were a must despite Father disliked eating vegetables and fruits. However, he would sometimes order food he suddenly got an appetite for, asking Mother and Sam to do him a favour.

Mother would sometimes complain to us that once the food Father specially asked them to make was out, his appetite would all of a sudden change, with him telling her nay. Conceivably, it would pose not a few problems between them. Every time, when Mother made such complaints to us, we would just laugh, saying Father was funny. Again, not realizing whether this phenomenon normal or not, we just did not want to play up it lest Father should find himself with problems in recovery that would only be seen as detrimental.

At the very beginning, when we four siblings sought a doctor and hospital for Father, John had searched over the Internet, attempting to find the information of the illness Father unluckily developed on one hand, and on the other, he had painstakingly searched for the information about the surgery Father had to take. Some information said the recovery could easily take a patient half a year or more, and during the whole process of the recovery, different patients would manifest different phenomena, including sudden changes in appetite. Problems about excretion would also be a distraught issue depending on the situation of different patients' speed of recovery. Therefore, it would be hard to say which belonged to normal or which belonged to the contrary. Thus and so, finding out Father's actual situation would have to wait for the coming body check-up two months later in Dr Chu's clinic.

Besides mah-jong, Father had one more hobby—horse race. He enjoyed watching the horses trot gracefully and run frantically with speed on an immense broad plain of grass more than anything relating to the theme of horse race. He was mesmerized in watching the horses more than in making bets, wisely thinking betting on animals was like ploughing the sand. Every time, he just bet a little as participation. Knowing Father had such a hobby as we did, we had once or twice taken him to the racecourse to see if it could also be one of our gatherings, and we found the answer absolute.

Every time in the racecourse, Father would enjoy watching the view along with the horses slowly walking on the tracks as their warm-up before the races started. When the races began, he would concentrate, putting his body and mind in one, on how the horses ran at full fling to compete with one another to gain the championship. What the word he described the scenes the horses competed in were 'breathtaking'. No matter if he won or lost, he would only say 'Dynamite, dynamite!' to the horses he admired much.

Since Father was terribly ill, we had not gone to the racecourse for almost a year. Undeniably, all of us longed to visit such a fantastic place after having missed it for so long, and when we asked Father about it, 'Of course, why not,' was his explicit reply to us.

With Father's firm reply, in two shakes, we arranged a day convenient for all of us to have an adventure there. Admittedly, we did not exactly have the same the attitude Father held—we like betting far more than watching the views or the horses as he did. That is our major difference, albeit, it did not make us have any dissent; we got along with each other more than well.

November 4, a Sunday, every one of us could enjoy this public holiday to the utmost, we thought. Thus and so, we nailed it down after all of us were on all fours about it. Father, no exception, agreed with the date we chose with a smile and a nod. We observed that he had more confidence this time we arranged the function than the last time he had. Concededly, after experiencing the feast we had at the restaurant last time, he had gained back not a little confidence. Yeah, success boosts confidence, and vice versa.

There were still ten odd days in the coming up of the event of the racecourse function we planned. Father kept on doing everything he could to make further progress in the recovery of his fragile body after undergoing operation twice. Every day, he kept both a peaceful and joyful mood, acting like a normal person and doing everything he wanted. Among what he did, eating appeared to be his great treat. Mother and Sam sometimes reported to us that Father always called for food, saying he was very hungry with his eyes opened wide and staring at them. Anyway, they said Father's this expression would sometimes make them scared. Was Father's situation normal or not? Again, we could not know.

The big day came, finally.

The racecourse, a place located in Sha Tin, occupying part of Hong Kong's precious territory with an immense plain of greenish grassland glutted with overwhelming views aiming at stunning everybody who comes. Every week, there are two horse races, except for months of vacation in extreme hot summer for horses so the horses can have a yearly rest. People can easily get there by taking the Mass Transit Railway with a stop provided there.

As soon as you admit through the entrance of the racecourse, all of a sudden, you will be unconsciously and uncontrollably attracted by the views there and eagerly take out your cameras or cell phones to pose everywhere. In a minute, you will even forget the real aim of the visit is to bet instead of considering it a day of sightseeing. Doubtless, it is a pleasant place for a family gathering to eat and take pictures in addition to making bets on horses. Not only do the locals like to come for entertainment—the people from every corner of the world also make it a tourist attraction and rendering Hong Kong, such a small place, no less popular and famous than a big country.

As we are members of the racecourse club, we are entitled to enjoy a discount in booking tables for their delicious buffet located on its top floor with stunning view. This time, as usual, we reserved a table, as Father had once or twice said he liked the buffet there.

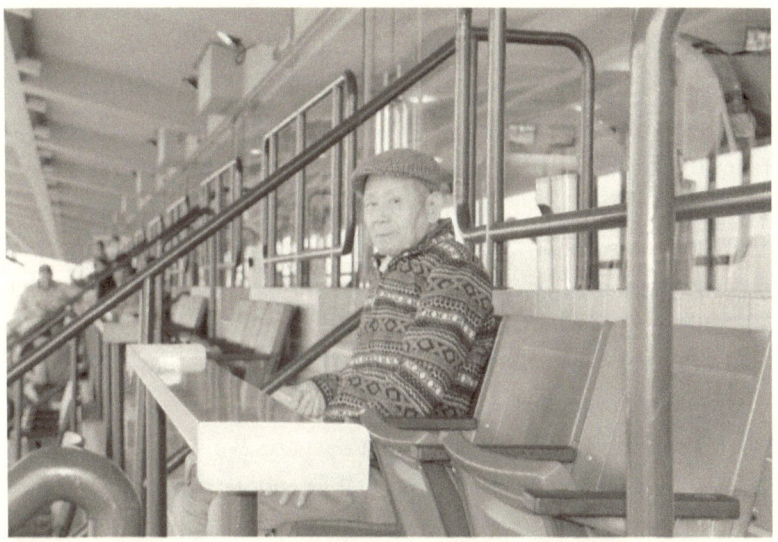

We arrived far earlier before the first race started in order to have food and gain time to study the races the club would be going to hold. Father looked well in both physical and mental shape, walking with normal paces to get food that the buffet served. Mother said they only took a little congee this morning to save space in their stomachs needed for the buffet. We laughed.

As to this activity, Father looked forward to eating and viewing. He only made a little bet on the horses he liked. When we looked back some months ago, when he was painstakingly doing everything more than he could to hopefully cope with the difficulties the recovery in the critical stage after magically surviving the first operation, we had not dared to think the day would really come of us seeing him able to do everything he wanted as before. This time was his first time to come to the racecourse since he had been ill. We could sniff out that he felt touched, and we were no less touched than he was. Instead of revealing such sentiments to each other, we kept it in our hearts, revealing another kind of feeling: happiness.

When every race started, Father used to go outside and sit on the bench the stand provides watching the horses running and competing with one another. One glance we captured from him was when he was like thinking, sitting there to wait for the race started. We took a picture of him. Father was not a talkative person, nor was he an active one. He liked silence—such silent that he was somehow a bit elusive. It was not easy to find out what he thought, not to mention prying about his inner world. Whenever we asked him what he thought, he would just say nothing. So independent a soul to bear by so old a man—we could not but be proud of him.

Usually there are ten races in a day, and we used to see them all before going home in the past. The whole function in a day would take us nearly ten hours, including taking transportation; and this time, there were reasons to worry if Father could stand all. Hence, after several races, we asked him if he would like to go home or stay. 'Oh, it is good. I am comfortable.' He replied to us again with a slight smile and nod. A slight smile and nod, such a welcoming expression, became a symbol of Father, though we could not remember when it began.

In fact, it began long ago, only we had not taken him seriously enough to notice it or feel it.

Curiously, life can find ways to teach us how to treasure the things around us that we may forget to treasure or even notice when it exists. Many times, it is a bit late!

Father had taken several rounds of the food the buffet served and ate not a little. He said to us the food was good and he had enough. We saw him sometimes walking to the washroom on his own without us accompanying him or approaching the counter to make bets—everything he once had done there in the past. He liked the place and enjoyed everything there, and he constantly lingered and lingered around. He was that simple, knowing how to appreciate things and seeing them as godsends. That was his unique way of living, and he had provided us a very good example to follow.

Unlike him, what we aimed for there was to win the races as many who came did. Whenever we lost, we would cry out or at least blamed or appeared unhappy. With Father as our example, we have learned the way of appreciating things around us as he did. Therefore, most of the time, we would keep a grip on ourselves by not going overboard. We thought we are more than blessed enough to have a man so simple and wise to be our Father to allow us room to find mantras about life. We sometimes even thought that Father was like a book with no sound but words intelligible enough to teach us how to live the simplest and happiest. He did this by revealing the least (*or even none*) of the dark sides of human nature, with as much love as possible to others and, in particular, to our every truly loved ones.

Humans are unluckily born with not a few experiences of the dark side of human nature. Nevertheless, we are simultaneously, luckily born with love enough that we are able to bring it into full play to dissolve these dark experiences.

Eventually, ten races finished. As a result, we lost rather than won, and we saw it was only to be expected. We laughed and headed home. The scenes with comments or even scolding which are full of foul words roaring by the people on this race or that race are commonplace at racecourses when they are emptying after the show, and we are no strangers to this typical phenomenon. However, we have been, every time, in a class by ourselves. This time, we exchanged our feelings with each other before discussing when we would come again, with cheers. Father responded to us several times with a slight smile and nod. We could feel his content—he was a lot more contented than after winning a considerable sum of money in bets. What we felt at that very moment was more than happy and blessed. Again, Father successfully and cheerfully experienced an outdoor function. We could not be happier and prouder.

Father's actual situation now was acting exactly like a normal person, except that there was a bag slapping on one side of his waist for urine excretion. Luckily, this posed no problem on him at all. What he showed us about it was that he saw it as saving time, without him spending time in the washroom about peeing. Although smacking of not a little cynicism, it was full of wisdom. Such is the wisdom that teaches us a way of getting rid of redundant sadness when encountering difficulties or changing, we grasped.

Three weeks later, Father would have a body check-up in Dr Chu's clinic again. By then, we would be sure if Father had successfully completed the recovery, restoring him to good health from the two operations performed on him half a year ago, with one substantial and risky.

These three weeks, Father behaved the same as he used to be, acting not a bit worried about the coming check-up. He was confident about it, we thought.

CHAPTER FOUR

The appointment made. Father woke up a bit earlier than usual in the morning to have himself gear up. We had arranged a van in advance to take us between places since we found it always convenient when it was hard to seek a taxi on the streets. The first stop would be a restaurant to have our morning tea with Chinese dim-sum Father favoured.

In the restaurant, Father ate what we ordered and drank the tea he liked. He ate and drank without much talking with us. We could not know why. We just thought he might be nervous to see Dr Chu, not knowing if he could again pass the check-up like last time. There were no two ways about it: the check-up this time was crucial. It would inexorably tell if Father had successfully recovered from the operations and, at the same time, tell if Father was bona fide restoring his health to normal with everything inside his body working well. Hence, it could be explained why Father would appear a bit nervous. We kept ordering food to eat and chatting with each other lest Father should discover that we had found his silence in question. As silent as he was, Father would on occasion utter words of good taste to us, referring to the food he ate. In return, we would say 'Eat more' to him.

To all intents and purposes, Sam and mother had once reported to us that Father, these ten-odd days, remarkably ate less than he did in the past. Nevertheless, we preferred seeing it normal lest Father should find us worried. Instead, we monitored

him a bit closer, seeing if there were other problems occurring
to him. The result was he was largely the same as he used to be,
except that he was eating less.

Owing to the body check-up that would come soon, we chose
to wait for it to verify Father's health and not to wrongly guess
without evidence supporting, which would unnecessarily make
him worried.

The tea finished, we accompanied Father to see Dr Chu.

Dr Chu greeted us with a smile and a gesture offering us
each a seat. After some regular and casual examinations over his
body, Dr Chu asked Father how he was doing. Father replied to
him that the question of excessive excretion remained, causing
him to excrete sometimes more than ten times a day. Dr Chu
replied to Father that it would depend heavily on each patient's
speed of recovery, and it would be hard to say if it was normal
until after finishing the check-up. Upon saying this, Dr Chu
guided Father into another room to have a thorough check-up
by scanning, which would precisely tell if Father's redundant
excretion in question was normal or not.

We waited outside and prayed and prayed by linking our arms
together, with our eyes tightly shut, hoping Father could pass the
check-up like last time, with the blood test showing the lowest
rate of cancer. We thought if it really happened, Father would
have really recovered from operations and would be progressing
well, with everything inside his body good and normal. It would
be more than rousing not only to Father but also to us. Then, the
days he would have would be at least easy after he had endeavoured
tremendously in confronting everything he had to face against
the deadly illness the past half year. We adamantly insisted that
Father deserved this, hoping the gods we prayed to could hear
our prayers.

Father and Dr Chu came out.

We sat with eyes barely brave enough to look at them coming out, perceiving them each wearing *a long face*, a lot different from last time they did. Our hearts uncontrollably beat far quicker, not knowing what exactly the check-up told. We were asked to come forward to listen to Dr Chu, and at that very moment, when we were being told the *harshest* and *cruellest* news by Dr Chu that Father's cancer had come back, none of us could remain unruffled but all burst into tears.

We were shocked. Dr Chu was shocked. He said he found out from the scanning that there was a new tumour growing fast and fiercely in Father's anus. He said he could not believe what he saw when he found the tumour unexpectedly growing that fast and fiercely. It was a rarity. We could tell he was speechless about it. Not knowing anything to say that would make Father feel better, we kept silent. We just listened carefully to Dr Chu, desperately hoping he would say he could still cure him. Without disappointing us, Dr Chu suggested a prompt operation to Father with full explanation on it. Father listened and nodded, acting the calmest one among all of us.

Our hearts were broken into fragments, triggering an outpouring of weeping in grief, being totally at our wits' end and not knowing what to say and do. We took Father's arms, holding his hands warmly and tightly, telling him not to be afraid and promising him he had us together to confront and battle the illness. Father nodded without a smile. We all cried except him. We really could not know how he could be that strong. His penchant for the greatest strength shown was out of his *love*—he knew once he cried, we would all go messy, and he did not want it to happen. He painstakingly bore his tears with only one aim—to save our tears to the utmost.

Entering the van and driving back home, we found there was a sudden dead silence terribly dominating the core of the van that we wanted to get rid of. To avoid such dead silence continuing to take hold and to swing the atmosphere, we asked the driver to turn on the music CD. In a minute, we were like in protest, filling the van with at least some sound. When humans recognize ourselves to be vulnerable to music, we found that music would be effective when played. With the soft melodies of the song wafting, we did feel a little better, finally able to begin finding subjects to talk about. Nevertheless, we could not find one suitable with our confused minds. What we did then was all the same holding tightly Father's hands, assuring him and consoling him with facial expressions. Hardly could we utter even a word about the operation Dr Chu prompted. Rather, we chose to find a right time to talk about it later to gain each other a while of composure that we all found we needed at that moment.

It was a *thunderbolt*—such was a thunderbolt that made us all fall apart at the seams!

'What went wrong?' We could not but think exceedingly. What had gone wrong between last time's body check-up to this time's, when the result of last time was so satisfactory? On earth, what had gone wrong in these stupid days? We could not help but think and think crazily and insanely.

Knowing we were unable to have time to trace back or ask or blame or whatsoever we would try to think of the reasons would be the cause, we chose to strain every nerve to act positively and optimistically to fight the battle with Father. Really, more often than not, life does not have many choices for us.

Back home, the first thing Father did was lay in the bed to take a rest. Since all of us had our own families in our hands, we said goodbye to him and left before telling him that we would be beside him always and asking him not to think too much for the time being.

Another piece of bad news ruthlessly stuck us the following day. We heard Mother say that Father would not want to have any kind of treatment at the hospital any more, saying he was sure that he was too fragile now to stand any operation. He added that he would not want to die in an operation room, saying the place was too *cold* and *lonely*. He asked us not to worry about him. Mother continued, saying that Sam had asked Father if he would trust some herbs effective against cancer some zealous people posted wholeheartedly over the Internet, aiming at helping sufferers. Father nodded and said, 'It might be the only way. Give it a shot so.'

Cold and lonely, it was conceivable that Father might not be afraid of death. He only wanted to have us all beside him when he was at that moment. We could tell how much he had immensely suffered mentally and emotionally the last two operations in such a place he described as cold and lonely.

Sam, at that point, searched over the Internet at full fling against the clock, hoping there would be herbs curing Father's new tumour. Efforts of a night and a day's searching awarded him five herbs, with each having a full explanation indicating how it would help keep the tumour in check or make it keep stable or even shrink. The user also had methods taught how to make the five components, in turn acting on the patient to bring about an ideal result. The whole treatment would take long. Father not only had to bear the extreme bitterness of the herb but also had to survive the unknown reaction inside the body it might cause.

It still sounded not bad if the herbs could work. Father could live without undergoing operation that would risk failure or worse owing to his fragility. That would be an alternative, we thought.

Without a better choice, Father took the herbs Mother boiled for hours in a kitchen so small that every corner of the house was rife with the pungent smell of it.

We did not know if he was too fragile to stand the herbs or there were other reasons, but Father *vomited* shortly after taking it.

We began worrying about the situation Father was. Should the herbs in question continue despite Father's response? We were like at a crossroads, desperately hoping for an indication guiding us which direction to go. We were actually in a fix—and such was a fix that made us all feeling immensely distraught.

Apart from vomiting, Father, at the same time, lost most of the appetite he had before after continuing to take the herbs. Every meal, he just had a little food. It was such as to render us unbearable. We rapidly came to think of abandoning the herbs, shifting to making the decision of trusting Dr Chu again. Nevertheless, it was merely our thought. We literally heard from Mother that Father would not take any operation at the hospital anymore. Should we just respect his thought or speak to him our thoughts? After struggling and struggling, we finally decided to find way to speak to him.

We went home together with a mission—convincing Father to receive the operation Dr Chu prompted. Our plan was, lunch first, and then a mah-jong game if Father found himself able to play with us, hoping the sound of mah-jong would create a climate to open up the topic that was unwelcome. Although he was badly uncomfortable, Father gave us a passionate reception when we got to him, saying nothing could be happier than seeing us. Before playing mah-jong, we had already sniffed out that he had to go to the washroom profusely within just an hour's time when we were having lunch and chatting. What's more, he ate poorly but vomited terribly. Eventually, we found ourselves unable to wait in persuading him about the urgent need of the operation we thought he in no way could flee.

'Father, if the herbs do not work, you have to go to the hospital and receive a cure before it is too late,' we said to him holding his hands tightly, hoping he would grasp us. 'We know it is hard for you to again to undergo an operation, but the reality is so. We really don't have any other choice,' we continued, making our gentle persuasion. 'The situation can be when one day you cannot get up of bed, you will be eventually sent to the hospital, so it is just a matter of time. However, it will pose a striking difference. If you go to the hospital in good time, you will stand a chance to receive a cure, but if you do it in the last moment, the case will only be pessimistic. We do not think you deserve the latter when you have made a lot of effort in the last half year. You do not have to be concerned about the matter of money. We can afford it. Even if we cannot, we will find ways out. How can we not cure you because of money? It is a crime—such a crime that opposes every instinct in our body.' We gently explained to him, looking him in the face.

Father was uninsured, working as a chef in the old time, without pension after retiring being in the vestiges of the kind of exploitation at that time. In those days, it was commonplace to lack of a piece of legislation fair enough to protect workers' welfare. Hence, we had to settle all the costs of his cure out of pocket. When we four siblings helped share the cost, he might think the money we spent had already gone down the drain, and he did not want to repeat it, so he gave up treatment, which he knew would only cost again considerably. Additionally, Mother is a rather money-minded person, and she might have said something in terms of money to Father, making him have such a worry. About it, we indeed had heard her gripe once or twice as proof. Mainly, she was complaining about the high cost of the surgery fees of the doctor and the exorbitant charges of every item of the hospital.

Inevitably, every house has its own problem. Ours is no exception.

Father showed us a countenance more in peacefulness than in sorrow. He tenderly said to us that all had done more than amazing in the past half year, and he was not going to take any kind of treatments suggested at the hospital. He explained to us that he did not have confidence enough to stand the operation, not to mention the strength required in recovery afterwards. He said he felt more than blessed to die old on his soft and warm bed with a wife and four loving children beside him. He then added, 'The laws of life dictate so. What more could I ask for when I am already so blessed?' Denoting we should not take everything for granted. 'I have enough, more than enough,' Father satisfactorily said to us, letting loose our hands that held him tightly and shifting to gently pat our faces and shoulders with a smile. 'Don't worry too much about me, good sons and good daughters.' He completed the conversation. Then he stood up and headed to the sitting room, turning on the television.

Although what he said all adhering to reason, it was flat-out heartbreaking.

This time, we saw our mission fail. The cause was we chose to respect what Father thought and insisted. We did not want to force him.

A week went by. Father had taken few more times the herbs Sam searched from the Internet.

The result was far worse than earlier. It was such as to render Father incapable of taking it anymore. Ironically, he took the herbs without choice in the first place and at last gave it up without choice either.

No herbs, no other remedies—we thought we could not see Father let it go at that. We began to not only worry but also *rush*. We saw a frantic endeavour in persuading him to receive treatment at the hospital was what we had to do at once brooking no delay. We went home again, hoping this time, when Father's situation was so bad that our persuasion would do the trick.

Father appeared far weaker than the last time we saw him. Apparently, not only did the herbs fail to work but also vastly worsened the inner functions of his body in a way. He could just speak in a low voice, with eyes telling us he was badly uncomfortable. Never did Father play up things. He used to keep a low profile in every spectrum in his life. Even when his life was in peril, like this moment, he still did not favour exaggerating. He let alone us to suggest him anything this time. When we opened up the topic of him receiving the operation, he reacted with an immediate response by nodding his head to attempt to save our breath.

With Father's nod, we called Dr Chu asking him to make arrangements to Father and then we made a call to the hospital asking them to reserve Father a room.

Today was December 9, a Sunday, and the appointment made was the following day. Therefore, we went home to see Father, aiming to stay with him to give him support and love in preparation for the following day's admittance to hospital. Tomorrow would be the third time he would go to hospital, and it was conceivable that he would feel hard. Understandably, no one wants to stay at a ghost-like place.

Father asked us to play mah-jong with him, and we were more than happy to do so when he still had mood and strength in doing it. While we played, Mother prepared us some fruits—grapes. Father, appeared to have an appetite enough to take the grapes out of the blue, eating them as delicacies when he all along has had not much interest in fruits. He looked good today. We smiled.

Without finishing four rounds to complete east, south, west and north of the game, Father shivered, saying he had to go to bed with some layers of blankets. Mother then told us that Father was that physically unstable lately by appearing good at one time and bad at another. We placed Father on the bed with a rather thick layer of blanket to keep him warm. Anyway, he still shivered, and he vomited a lot later. All the grapes he ate before had he thrown up. Not knowing what virtually happened to his inner body, Sam helped him measure blood pressure, only to find the result showing his state terribly unstable and abnormal. Sam suggested Father go to the hospital straight away lest at night Mother should not know what to do if he got even worse.

Father nodded again.

A day earlier than the appointment made, Father went to the hospital for safer conditions where he could have professional medical care, which home could not provide him.

Although we could rest physically for a while, we dared not take anything about Father lightly but stayed vigilant. Truly, all of us felt hemmed in by affliction appearing shattered—inside out.

'Fear not but confront' was our pledge and new motto that propped us up when life was encountering such grim a challenge as ever. The only way to answer such a challenge was so, we insisted.

CHAPTER FIVE

Again sent to the hospital, Father chose to behave in his old ways, acting as if nothing it was big but showing as much humour as he could. Once admitted, the nurses greeted him, saying hello indicating to him a sign of their recognition. We told Father that they could recognize him, and Father replied to us with a sarcastic smile that it was better not to know this kind of people, not to mention the recognition of them. We laughed a lot to support his view.

A series of check-ups seemed to have posed no problems on Father. He let the nurses do anything to him without him asking what they did. Clearly, he knew well all of the procedures before operation. Again he said with a wry smile to us that it was better not to have known a bit of them, not to mention being familiar with them. Despite Father speaking only so little, we found his words full of axioms. Father was elite, in a briefer way, to speak of life, making us find any further explanation about what he said merely superfluous every time. We responded to what he said with a chuckle as well as a mixed feeling that was hard to reveal.

Dr Chu had explained explicitly to us that this time he would remove the new tumour located in Father's anus, saying he could not believe it growing so fiercely and fast. Before the operation, Father had to undergo a thorough scanning through MRI (magnetic resonance imaging) to see if the cancer had spread to another area of his body. If, unluckily, the cancer had spread, Dr

Chu might call off the operation. Thus, the scanning tomorrow morning would be critical. The result of it would pin hope or dash hope on Father's destiny.

Hence, we prayed and prayed, hoping the result of the scanning would come out good to let Father at least get a chance to receive the operation. As to the operation, we realized that one more miracle would have to happen to Father again like the first time he received the substantial and risky one. Undoubtedly, we needed that miracle again! We hoped such miracle would be glutted with sympathy and forgiveness of our greed, take his side as he had once made a mammoth effort in confronting the illness and would be *willing* to do so again.

Dawn cracked, wakening most of the people to work or study. We, with no exception, had our jobs to provide us a living. Still, we went to see Father, making time as best we could. Today, Father looked nice, telling us he had undergone the scanning in the morning and waited for the result that would come out tomorrow. We responded to him by lifting up our thumbs, denoting the result would only be good as we wished. Father smiled and nodded.

Father had ordered a meal for his lunch. Seeing him with appetite to take food, we were much relieved. When asked what he had ordered, Father appeared serious, with eyes opened wider than usual, saying he had ordered a bowl of congee with meat, adding he did not want the congee to be too bland like Mother made. When the congee came, he even put some salt onto it. Clearly, he wanted to bring out his appetite with a rather tasty flavour. We supported him, saying he could eat whatever he found fit for his stomach. Father not only nodded and smiled but also said 'Of course' referring to what we said to him.

He could eat the meal well and prepared what to order for the dinner in the evening, looking at the menu and choosing.

He must have forgotten he had an operation tomorrow morning and had to stop taking food right then and took the laxative to empty his bowels. Once he got it, he did not get angry or disappointed but grinned and bore it with nods. When the nurse brought him the laxatives and instructed him to take them, he signalled us to leave, meaning he would be busy soon. The matter of fact was he did not want us to see him feeling hard with the effect of the laxative taken. Undeniably, it was love we could not but extol—how love plays a role in our lives when facing a hard time, especially when being totally in a predicament.

In the past half year, at the time staying at the hospital, Father used to conceal the most painful scenes occurring to him from us to the utmost, leaving himself alone to swallow every bit of the pain and goriness without letting us see. The way he adopted was trying his best to make himself look all right or at least not the worst every time in front of us to keep us from over worried or scared. It was evident that it was no easy task. We did not know how he could make it. For a certainty, he was a bona fide strong man. A strong man with deep and silent feelings inside him that would easily make the people around feel touched. Yeah, Father was contagious in terms of sentiment.

We went home after saying goodbye to Father and told him that we would come tomorrow morning to give him support.

Night would go regardless of whether you can sleep or not. Morning came, and I could barely open my eyes, finding myself laid awake and spending the whole night worrying. For the third time, in the morning found David and me going to the hospital to *support* Father before a surgery. It was afflicting, albeit we geared ourselves up to face it. Within an hour, we arrived at the hospital as we promised Father the previous day, thanking to the smoothness of the traffic.

When we arrived, Father was sitting in a wheelchair, already heading to the operation room, pushed by a hospital worker. As bare as it could be, we could still see him in good time, when he was waiting for a kind of designated lift that transports patients from wards to operation rooms. Father smiled at that very moment upon seeing us, saying to me and David that John and Sam had not yet arrived. There might have been some alteration about the time of the operation without our knowledge, getting a head start for about half an hour. On the point of sending Father into the lift, Sam and John appeared in time, incentivising Father not a little. The worker, in two shakes, let us talk with Father without going straight into the lift.

Father smiled and nodded, saying he would come out to see us and asked us not to worry. In return, we said as many nice words as we, at that moment, could think of to him, asking him not to fear. In transience, Father disappeared with the closing door of the lift he took.

The operation was to take an hour or more.

As we waited, we whiled away the time by taking breakfast together at the canteen the hospital provided. When we entered, we found the canteen renovated. Suddenly, a mixed feeling hardly explained occurred to us. We remembered that the very first time when we took breakfast here was half a year ago, when Father underwent his first time in life the biggest operation and miraculously survived. It was hard to believe he was now in the operation room again to battle the cancer after, for months, making a great deal of endeavour to suffer and confront the pain in recovery with patience and endurance.

It was goddam ironic that when it would have been time for us to bask in the success of the recovery Father painstakingly made, it was not what was happening. Inexplicably, life will be somehow decorated with backfire. And such is the backfire that will, in a way, make our lives more legendary.

We could find that the expression Father showed then was apparently nowhere near confident like the past two times, meaning he might have lost faith in trusting medicine with his ferocious illness. We knew he just barely gave the operation a hope that he could not but embrace.

When I had no idea about the result of the scanning Father took yesterday morning, John told me about it as we took our breakfast.

It was as *a bolt from the blue* when I heard John say Father's cancer had not only come back but also spread.

John said Dr Chu called him in the morning, explaining the result of the scanning and saying Father's cancer had already spread to the liver and a little bit to the lung. He said the operation would be all the same going on, promising us that he would do his level best to cure him. As to what he would or could do, he said it could only depend on the situation when the operation was underway, which was critical to Father's life and death. John concluded that Dr Chu still could not precisely tell us what he would do in the operation.

Seeing me appear so stifled upon getting exposure to such a bad news, John stopped for a while to let me find ways to breathe. With consolation, he talked again, saying for now we might only have Dr Chu to trust.

My feeling was somehow a bit emotional with such a hit. Did it mean Father's cancer was incurable? How could it be so brutal? Would Father have to suffer more and more pain? Would the cancer in his liver grow fast and fiercely? How long would Father still have? Was the cancer going to kill him without mercy? Mainly, was it a joke to have him go through far more than he could in confronting the illness in the past several months only to get another cancer? If so, where did the logic and reason lie? At a stroke, a mountain of such radical questions stuck my brain, making me fail to utter a word. To avoid the words coming out destructively when I was so angry, I kept my head, trying to find ways to talk again.

Finally, I could find my tongue by uttering some whispers responding to what John said to me. Seeing me having calmed down a bit, John further explained to me about Father's situation with the information he searched from the Internet. He said the cancer could be said the deadliest and worst, and what we could do was to make Father happy and easeful in the remainder of his time. He hoped Dr Chu could successfully remove the new tumour located in Father's anus first and then find another remedy to treat the other areas. I nodded to him, saying yes.

Soon, John sighed, explaining to us that the speed of liver cancer can grow much faster than that of others and will cause the patient a lot of pain. Once it grows fast, it will pose an immediate threat on the sufferer's life, causing immense pain and, at last, a coma. The period can be as short as just few months or even less. Subsequently, John seemed not to know what to say about it. Paused a little, he again talked. Sam listened to what he said, appearing a tattered face. Nobody could bear such a bad news. We were all heartbroken.

All along, looking at the bright side has led us to not a few successes, we see these are the literal fact we should not ignore. This time all the same, we should not ignore or forgot it just because of setbacks. We, again, as we used to be in the past, looked at this time's worst hit in a positive, optimistic way in order to not missing any miracle that would happen to Father.

When there is a will, there is a hope. Only with hope can life go on its way without swerving from its route.

Embracing hope and harbouring positive attitude was one thing, what was more important and realistic was to act in chorus to not only support Father but also to make him live happily. We came up with an idea not to let Father know the whole truth of the illness looming over him. Only so could he live without worries and fears to reach a normal and happy life.

On the other hand, we began to look back in the past few months, hoping there were clues we could find if there was anything that went wrong. Among us was Sam, who took care of Father the most. He began to talk. He said Father did appear a bit anomalous especially for the past few weeks. Sometimes Father would open his eyes wide, staring at the food placed on the table prepared by Mother and him, asking him what kinds of food those were, like suspecting what he would be going to eat. Sam said Father did not seem to believe the food he was going to eat was decent enough but bad making him sick. In the morning, he would appear exceedingly hungry, looking at the two big boiled eggs that he was going to eat with some enigmatic smile, saying the eggs were amazing. Sam said he and Mother would be scared with such an expression he unwittingly showed sometimes. Adding he had no idea of such phenomenon wanted to tell them. Anyway, most of the time, Father appeared normal.

John came to suspect the eggs, saying there might be so much protein that Father could not take it all but it was absorbed by the new tumour. He argued that protein might be favourable to cancer. He said owing to this theory, it could explain why the cancer would recur to Father in so short a time, growing so fiercely and fast. For an octogenarian, two big eggs each morning may be in excess in terms of protein absorption, not to mention for a person who had cancer before. Protein may pose a greater danger of recurring cancer when it is too much to absorb more than any other nutrition in the food. At the same time, it can also explain why Father would love eating the eggs so much. It was horrible! It could mean the power of cancer was outrageous! He said it might be our carelessness.

John then again searched the Internet, attempting to probe into the mystery of the relevance of food and cancer.

We crumbled hearing the news of Father's cancer not only recurring but also spreading. We could not but try to do everything we could think of to find a way for Father's remaining days to live the longest and happiest as possible.

John talked again. He said some information through Internet told us that a patient with cancer needs protein to help recover after operation. It is because protein can enhance the human immune system, our frontline ability to fight disease. Without contracting or getting other diseases by absorbing enough protein, a patient can recover ideally without obstacles. It makes sense. The thing is, if the protein is in excess, it will be favourable to the new tumour. Still, it is a mystery to prove what makes the new tumour develop in the first place. It could not be protein, or no one will dare to take any food with it. That is to say, Father might have stored some of the hidden cells of cancer inside his body that could not be tested or scanned in the first body check-up, making us and Dr Chu believed that the cancer was gone. Without us knowing it still clandestinely existed, the cancer had never gone. Only it was so wily that it could hide.

We thought if food was so crucial to a cancer patient after operation, Dr Chu should have advised us about it. We remembered that when Father had finished the first operation, we could not wait to ask him what Father could eat or best eat to benefit his recovery and keep the cancer in check. Dr Chu replied to us only that if Father liked the food, he could eat all kinds of food. We took what he said seriously, letting Father eat whatever he wanted. To all intents and purposes, what the food Father ate was largely wholesome. Even if the two big boiled eggs may be excessive in protein that Father might not absorb all, it hardly would be the culprit of the new tumour. Therefore, we gave up blaming the eggs, but positively, we found recipes conducive to a cancer patient's recovery instead.

We knew we didn't have any time to think of the past but to think of the coming days what we could do to Father the best in terms of not just taking care of him but also finding him suitable food. John went on surfing the Net and came to learn that a cancer patient can try foods that are more alkaline than acidic. It says lemon water is one that wonderfully works wonders. He laughed, saying it was a piece of cake to make a glass of lemon water—why would we be so late to do it? He then added that we had to make Father drink two to three glasses of it a day afterwards. He then said with some sardonic humour, 'No wonder a motto says, "If life deals you lemons, make lemonade," sarcastic enough!' As to some other recipes with medical properties especially against cancer, John found several easy-to-make soups that might suit Father as well.

Happily successful in searching for some results, we began to believe in food therapy and thought it would be an effective remedy against Father's illness.

Mother was still on the way, and we thought before she arrived, we had to spend a little time to arrange how to weigh our words in telling her the situation Father was in, to avoid too much triggering her emotions and feelings. John then suggested telling her Father's cancer had already spread and, after today's operation, there would be nothing more to do but to let him live as long and as happily as he could. He said Mother would understand what this meant. We decided to elude the word *irremediable* or words carrying similar meaning to her in the content.

Mother arrived, sitting down with a sigh and asking how long the operation Father had taken would be. It would be nearly more than an hour, we replied. Slowly, John began to talk to her about the result of the report of the scanning Father underwent yesterday morning. Surprisingly, Mother did not appear too shocked. She could talk, even talked more than us about it. She said it was only to be expected, saying Father, in this case, would not live long. She was calmer than we had expected. She thereupon asked us to go for lunch at a restaurant nearby—on one side to have lunch, and on the other to plan what to do.

At the restaurant, John displayed to Mother some of the recipes he found on the Internet that had medical properties conducive to Father's illness, and mainly, he asked her to choose some of them to prepare for him. However, she seemed not to be so zealous about it. She complained about how she was already exhausted with the toiling she had now at home in taking care of Father instead. Furthermore, she pointed out that our Father would not like these kinds of soup. 'So lemon water would be far easier to make,' John said, not stopping from persuading her. However, Mother remained unconvinced, saying Father would not like it either.

Sam then said he would make different kinds of fruit juices at his home, saying he could make it in the morning and then bring it to Father. Yeah, we thought we should do something to Father's illness instead of just letting it be. Since we found Mother appeared physically exhausted, we asked her if she would like us to employ a domestic helper to aid her. She replied to us saying no, explaining to us that she did not like a stranger staying with her at home.

When we were about to finish the lunch and go back to the hospital to see Father, John's mobile rang. He could not wait to pick it up, knowing it was Dr Chu with a glance to the screen displaying his phone number. We saw John calmly listen to what Dr Chu said to him on the phone, and within minutes, he put down the mobile and explained to us what Dr Chu had said to him about the operation.

John's countenance appeared a little bit off beam. He said Father's new grown tumour located in the anus had not removed. He quoted Dr Chu, telling us that Father's situation could not inspire any optimism. Since the cancer had already spread, he said it was futile and dangerous to remove the tumour located in the anus at this final stage. Doing so would only pose a potential threat on Father's life. He added that even if Father could get out of the jaws of death in the operation, he could hardly make a recovery given that the extensiveness of the cancer spread would relentlessly deteriorate his ability to do it. It would only culminate in a rather poor situation.

In that event, what Dr Chu had done in the operation, we could not wait to ask. John said he had reopened the artificial excretory opening he closed last time to let Father excrete the solid waste with a bag again carrying on his waist, hoping the excretion through the anus would decrease from a little to none afterwards. If it could work, Father would be a lot less afflicted than before of needing to excrete through anus more than ten times a day. Asked how long Father would still have, John said Dr Chu *promised* he would at least have half a year to nine months quality life if nothing serious happened to him in the intervening time.

Mother began asking questions. She asked John if Dr Chu had explained how the tumour located in the anus would further develop when it still existed. John said Dr Chu merely preferred it being there under Father's circumstances. Dr Chu had also said it would not grow any more without explicitly explaining to John how or why.

In fact, we all were in a mess—'not knowing what to do next' was an apt description of us.

All the same, we adamantly insisted that we should let Father live as happily as he could in the remaining time he would have. How to make him live the happiest was the thing we needed to rack our brains. At last, we came up with a plan and saw eye to eye with each other. As we all know, one can only live the happiest without worries and fears, so we thought if Father knew the actual situation he was in, by no means could he live the happiest. Such fearful living would only be a kind of prolonged ordeal.

Our plan was we would tell Father the least he needed to know, but not the whole. After making such a decision, we went back to the hospital to see him.

Father lay in the bed with consciousness, saying he was tired. We asked him to take a rest, telling him that his situation was all right. Father nodded with eyes half-closed, wanting a sleep desperately. We stayed for a while and left, leaving him to a band of professional nurses to attend to him.

The next day, we made time to see Father no matter how prolific our daily routine was. Father lay in the bed with eyes staring up at the ceiling, looking like he had questions to ask us. We greeted him good morning and asked after him. He replied to us that he was waiting for an operation. We were baffled, scratching our heads in front of him, and we said gently to him that he had already undergone the operation yesterday morning. He replied to us with a little confusion that this morning there was another one as well. We then said that there was none this morning, adding that the one he had undergone yesterday morning was good, and now he just needed to take enough rests to make recovery. He then nodded, saying he might have forgotten yesterday morning's operation. We found Father had already appeared some kinds of confusion with his train of thought.

Father was a person who never mixed up things with others. Once he got the answer from us, he would stop arguing or suspecting.

Asked if Dr Chu had said when he could eat, Father said he could eat whenever he wanted with words short and precise. We found that he began to appear a bit mistrusting Dr Chu. It was understandable. We laughed and showed him our consent asking him what he had ordered to eat for lunch. He said a bowl of congee with nice fish and meat plus a cup of Western tea with milk and sugar. As soon as we were talking about it, a worker brought him the food he ordered. Father smiled when the food came, saying he was hungry.

After the food placing elegantly on a smaller table that was movable around his bed, Father could effortlessly handle all things on his own without our help in making the food with its designated utensil neatly and conveniently ready to eat. As to etiquette, Father, throughout his life, used to behave at his most meticulous with his very presence suggesting humility and suaveness, making him no less than a learned man. We observed that he could only eat slowly despite him saying he was hungry. A bowl of congee took him a rather long time to finish. We accompanied him eating, asking him if the congee was tasty enough. He said it was not bad, commenting further that the flavour of fish was better than that of the meat. As to the tea, he just drank a little, saying it was not hot enough.

Yeah, Father only enjoyed the *hottest* drinks except beer.

Father had not asked us about his situation. Instead, we opened up such topic to him when we found the atmosphere a bit warmed up after he had taken some food. We told him that Dr Chu had reopened the closed artificial excretory opening on one side of his abdomen for his solid waste excretion. We explained to him that it would decrease the excretion through his anus gradually, and one day it would completely stopped. The operation done yesterday was for this. He had not asked if Dr Chu had removed the new tumour located in his anus or not. We, as well, keeping him from worrying too much and had not mentioned about it, saying what he needed now was to take rest. At last, we assured him by saying he would be all right and could completely recover day by day.

Although we had not lied to Father in saying the new tumour developed in his anus was gone, that could also be a lie when we had not told him it still existed. Nevertheless, we could not have a choice but did so because we wanted him to live his remaining days happily.

The coming festival—Chinese Tung Chee—would definitely be an incentive to encourage Father's mind and body to progress forward. Father liked Chinese festivals. He liked them mainly because there were always family gatherings. Given that, we attempted to lure Father to live in a happier mood by telling him that if he could get discharge from the hospital before Tung Chee, we would have dinner at a restaurant to celebrate it. Wonderfully, Father's eyes immediately shone, and he broadened his smile while exclaiming Tung Chee was around the corner. 'It is so quick, so quick!' He could not help saying. Without knowing what he exactly meant, we told him there were still ten days away and asked him to get a thorough rehabilitation at the hospital by staying a happy mood. Father then said it was so fast to live a year. We, at that moment, looked at each other, beginning to know what Father meant.

Father used to keep silent only, with words short and precise every time. Although he might seem difficult to read, he was virtually the one the easiest to figure out.

Spending time at the hospital was never for a minute an easy task, but even Father adopted a way of grinning and bearing through it. Every morning he was up with the lark, waiting. Waiting for the breakfast he had ordered, waiting for the lunch Mother would bring him, waiting for our individual turns to see him, waiting for the dinner before going to sleep. When, ruthlessly, some of the nights offered him different kinds of physical afflictions the illness brought, making him unable to sleep one wink, he waited for the morning to resume the same pattern of a day's routine called 'waiting'.

Owing to the operation run on him this time not causing severe physical damage, Father must have thought he could be discharged from the hospital soon, and we had heard him ask about it several times. What we replied to him was he had to take more and more rests to make his body strong enough to stay at home with Mother. Most of the time, Father used to offer us his tutored ears by taking all what we said to him without further ado, and this time, he acted the same. Conceivably, that was not only the love between us but also the trust.

Literally, Father needed great care taken under his de facto situation. We were afraid of Mother's inability in this area, which might make things worse. Mother is not young either, and the thing is she has had quite a few problems about her own health as well. What's more, she appeared reluctant to take in a domestic helper at home. Indubitably, our family could easily enter into an emergent state or even a crisis if we could not handle it well. Sometimes, some horrible pictures would be summoned up on our minds, like Father would suddenly need immense help at home sitting up or walking around and Mother would only stumble down when helping him. If the two fell to the floor with no one to provide urgent help in time, the situation would be lamentable. What if such a situation happened at midnight, we dared not think of the consequences that we all could not afford.

We discussed with Mother about our concern once. She seemed to have a plan herself. She said she did not like any strangers at home staying with her, refusing employing a domestic helper. Asked if she could be able enough to take care of Father, she replied to us that she would take care of him as best she could, adding she would only manage to do so when Father could, on his own, at least move and walk. If he became too weak to do so, she would suggest for him to stay at the hospital.

That seemed to be our consensus.

With such consensus, we at least knew what to do when Father appeared to be in the situation wherein Mother said she could not offer help.

Apart from strength, there may be a lot more one requires to have when it comes to taking care of a seriously ill patient. When such situation occurs to a couple, love and sacrifice would be certainly something indispensable they cannot lack. Would Father and Mother go through such a test, leaving each other the best chapter, with the greatest love storing in their memories as their best memories? Should we doubt that? We could not know. We could just hope for a consummate outcome. After all, they were a couple, only they themselves knew what they could give each other. Outsiders or even their children could hardly say anything of it.

When a couple has come a long way to become an old couple, it is already a blessing. Such is a blessing that tells them they should love each other even with sacrifice until the end to avoid regrets.

Father could eat well these several days at the hospital, except that he complained he was tired for nothing. Not exactly knowing what went wrong inside his body, we did not want to have it assessed in any way. We thought no assessment would come out good when Father's situation was like that. Instead, we talked to Father with some funny topics, attempting to divert some of the attention he had focused on his body. Like magic, Father could easily be distracted in talking with us with not a little humour as he did in the past.

When talking about the phenomenon, one episode he felt weird amused us a lot. Father said he felt weird finding people, with their whole body, sitting on the bed with the small movable table almost fully rotated tightly round the upper part of their body to eat. He said it was strange. Why not put their feet down the bed and eat with the table a bit distant from their body with ease? We asked if they were badly sick and could hardly do what Father found to be a bit proper, and he said he had seen them walk. 'Even faster than me,' he added. We burst into huge laughter, filling the room where before there was blatant silence. Father began to be fond of talking about what he saw at the hospital, quoting one incident after another to us with a great sense of humour. We, as soon as not, became his listeners, offering claps and roars as his rewards.

There was one we felt it even more amusing when Father said he found some doctors attending to their patients were actually for charging attendance fees. 'How are you today?' Such an endearment was their only words to their patients most of the time with nothing actually done to the patients before they left. When we asked him how he saw Dr Chu, Father said, 'The same, no difference. Every day he came to see me with "How about you today?" such an endearment with many times nothing actually done on me.' This time Father did not nod but shook his head with a wry smile.

Staying long at the hospital really could make Father see a lot that we could not see. Thus and so, listening to what Father said of the hospital's anecdotes became another kind of knowledge of life that we could not learn elsewhere.

One of Father's hands was as the previous two times embedding with a medical nutrition tube into a blood vessel to support his whole body strength and nutrition enough to stay alive, although he could take food. We could observe Father would sometimes take a serious look at that tube, wanting to ask it something seemingly. Whenever we spotted him and asked him what he wanted to know about it, he would reply to us by saying 'Nothing, just having a look.'

Presumably, he must have found that tube stupid in failing to make his stomach full and must have been looking forward to the day he could get rid of it. Yeah, we were sure of this day would come.

'The day after tomorrow is Chinese Tung Chee.' Father said with a slight smile. We all responded with excitement by saying yes and telling him that we had arranged a dinner at the restaurant we used to go to. 'Good,' replied Father. No one could firmly say to Father that he could get discharge from the hospital and joined the dinner with us. Father, as well, did not ask us about it but presumed he would also be in the dinner, asking us what we had ordered to eat. 'Eat whatever you want to.' We replied to him in unison in two shakes. 'Of course,' Father raised his voice a bit replying to us.

Subsequently, John called Dr Chu, consulting him whether Father could get discharge from the hospital in two days. Dr Chu said Father's situation could only be expected to not get worse too fast, asking us to take great care of him and let him live happily without worries. He said he could go home any time on condition that we could take care of him. With such a reply from Dr Chu, we jubilantly went to inform Father of it.

'Father, you can celebrate Tung Chee with us tomorrow.' We could not wait to tell him upon getting to him. 'Dr Chu said you can go home.' We added with not a little outburst emotion. We could not know why this time we would be so stirred. The reason might be we had concealed the awful truth about the actual situation from Father that Father would never know why we would do so. Yeah, it is painful to have a person not knowing why you would do something onto him when the reason is love that you cannot tell him. Therefore, we were not suddenly, but all along once since concealing the truth from him, stirred with different kinds of emotions.

Father, in return, appeared a lot more excited than we were. He said how much eager he, after staying at the hospital these ten days, had been to have a haircut. He asked John to arrange him time enough to visit a barbershop before going to the restaurant. 'No, no, I have to go home also to have a bath after finishing the haircut.' He added. Smiling broadened his mouth not a little, showing his enthusiasm in joining the dinner with us to celebrate Tung Chee, which many Chinese consider a festival an even bigger than Chinese New Year—Father was no exception. Father was a man who known for loving family gatherings, especially when they were Chinese Festivals. Truly, every time, such a gathering would bring us not a little happiness, making us understand in what way we should feel blessed and in what way we should love each other.

Father was in no ways a person who could draw crowds; nevertheless, obliviously, he could make us converge every time in all gatherings. Simultaneously, he would not step into the limelight in every gathering, but he could make all gatherings shine. This was absolutely his charisma that he brought into full play to the family he loved. We could not but heap praise and admire him so much. In fact, he had not done anything, and he just did everything without ado.

John, seeing Father appear like a child, could not wait to play. He found himself impelled to reply to him that he would arrange a van tomorrow for a whole day's transportation, meaning we could go anywhere Father wanted to. Father nodded. In the meantime, we found him unable to stop his excitement when we asked him to take rest. He said he had rest enough after lying in the bed for ten days, saying he could even go home now. 'I can walk, I can eat—there is nothing I am unable to do,' said Father with not a little pride. We then said yes to support him, praising him as our super father. We all laughed, drawing not a little attention from the neighbourhood in the meanwhile. They, as well, showed their sincerity to us in denoting our father great.

Seldom had Father demanded jobs from us like this time. He asked Mother to prepare him a suitable shirt and trousers for the dinner. He asked Sam to find him a nice traditional barbershop to let him also can have a beard cut there. He asked John to call Dr Chu if he needed to take any pills back home. He appeared more conscious than we were. When we looked at him as if inquiring him about his smartness, he said to us that he had thought about it for many days while lying in the bed to ease the monotony. He was not only smart but also positive and optimistic. Yes, we needed him this way. It was fabulous!

CHAPTER SIX

The big day came. Every one of us dared not to take anything lightly but stayed vigilant.

The first stop was to the hospital to pick up Father along with all his stuff he brought with him when the day he came in. It is always a phenomenon: a room is a lot more abundant with happiness when a patient leaves than when they come in. Once again, we were like on top of the world in taking Father out. It took us not much time in packing all the stuff. Within half an hour, we could get downstairs into the van we had arranged after paying the fees the hospital charged at the cashier counter.

Begun with not a little euphoria, we hoped today it would end in the same, or at least Father would have a joyous gathering with us whom he saw as pearls.

Father appeared no less excited to get into the van than we were. Deplorably, he started to vomit shortly after the van had travelled only some distance. John made a decision of calling off the stop at barbershop, realizing that Father possibly could not stand the haircut. Asked what he had eaten in the morning, Father said he had taken a sandwich and a cup of Western tea. No one could tell if the food or others made him vomit like this. We just could try our best to console him on one hand and on the other convincing him to go home to get some rest first. 'Go straight to the restaurant,' Father replied. 'I can get a rest there.

It would be okay. If we go home now, we would be very late to the restaurant then.' He went on saying. We did as Father said.

We all realized that Father would be afraid that once he was driven back home, he might not go to the restaurant then. He was desperate to go to the restaurant to join with us the big day we had buzzed about for a week. Such was the desperateness that told us he had attached a great deal of importance to us and the festival to such an extent that he had to give it a shot at any cost about his *fate*.

It was abundantly clear that what Father manifested to us was love—the greatest love on earth with no strings attached.

It was certainly a bold attempt when Father could not guarantee if he would vomit again. That he risked such an attempt showing how much he was eager to have happy moments with us this time, which he especially cherished. He just did not want to miss it. We continued taking the van. Father appeared a bit better than before. He had not vomited, at least, or he had already thrown up all he could. Arriving at the restaurant, we were ushered to a room reserved with a mah-jong table set the way it was every time we came. Father smiled, saying there would be more and more people coming tonight due to the festival, meaning it was good to have had a room reserved in advance. We all sat down first to have our favourite tea or drinks before going to the mah-jong table. Not knowing if Father wanted to play, we found we had to ask him about it first. When we were about to ask, Father was already in motion, standing up and moving towards the mah-jong table set. He was awesome!

Many say the roaring sound of mah-jong tiles falling on the table with one tile striking another can heal some ailments humans unluckily get for unknown reasons. Some even say no other cure is better and more effective than the cure of mah-jong. They play mah-jong mainly captivated by the sound of it more than other things. Undoubtedly, the ambiance when playing mah-jong can be abundantly riotous to make all the involved deeply concentrated. As a result, when they are paying full attention in playing it, they will forget all their worries and misgivings they have without any remedies prescribed. Some say mah-jong can even delay or prevent people from developing the symptoms of second childhood. Although there is not much evidence that can firmly substantiate the above-mentioned, the people who enjoy playing mah-jong do have a great moment to share with one another. In fact, most of the people playing this game seek fun rather than seek others as gamble.

Father's slow motion had revealed not a little of his frailty, which had us worried and heartbroken. More than obvious, he became weaker and weaker with the resurgent cancer. Reality is the inevitable thing in our lives and we can only *accept* and *face*. Seeing the way Father accepted things, we could not but feel ourselves inferior to him inside and outside. The reason we had not told him the cancer in his body had spread and was incurable was that we wanted him to be the way he was now. We did not want to have him any excessive untoward change. That was to say, we wanted him to live his remaining days the most positive and optimistic, and above all, the happiest and the most easeful.

Father did his utmost over the mah-jong table, attempting to prevent us from seeing him appear terribly fragile. He intended to divert our attentions from his poor health by acting as a great pretender. He played and played without asking to take five. In a sense, he might have enjoyed playing mah-jong a lot and did not want to miss such a chance to play with us in such a big day. We could see him appear more aggressive without respect to gauging his ability in doing it. For all his pains, he eventually called for a pause, asking Sam to accompany him to the washroom. He walked terribly slow, taking plenty of his strength to finish a step walking. With the sight of his shadow walking with Sam holding him tightly, at that moment, we all got a great intensity of feeling in our hearts, making us fail to even utter a word but keep awful silent instead.

At last, Sam took Father back home without having the dinner with us. It was conceivable that Father was exhausted and feeling very hard. Today, he had done far more than his ability allowed him to do by bringing out all his strength to take the van to the restaurant and play several games of mah-jong with us. He was superb, insanely superb!

At the dinner, we opened up the topic of taking care of Father to Mother, mainly with a view to seeing if she alone at home could do the duties for this task. It turned out that she appeared pessimistic more than optimistic, negative in preference to positive, indifferent rather than enthusiastic. She eventually did not hide but showed us the white feather in reference of it. She said she did fear, adding she had problems with her own health and saying she found it impossible to take care of a badly ill person at home. Asked if a domestic helper could help, she adamantly told us no. In this case, it would be increasingly hard to guarantee Father's safety at home. What would Mother want then? We pondered.

When we were racking our brains to find ways to solve problems, Mother seemed to elude all the questions she had to face but found ways to shirk. The way Mother acted now would only defy all possible solutions. We could not but begin to worry about Father's safety at home when he was now even too weak to take basic care of himself. Nevertheless, we chose to mollify Mother by commending her competent enough to take good care of Father if only she was not over afraid. 'Mother, you may not know you have, all along, already done very well. Never forget there are still us. Anytime we can offer help, should you fear nothing,' we added. However, she seemed not to be that confident as we wished; she was shaking her head constantly.

Only when something special imbued with life will it be different. It is already not that easy for a man and a woman to meet and love and to culminate in an old couple with children and grandchildren. If Mother could pluck up her courage a bit in taking care of Father with all her love, her life would definitely be embellished not a little with such special things collected into her memories which she could at any time recall as pearls with tears and joy. The significance of life owes much to this perspective. Unfortunately, Mother seemed to fail at grasping this important axiom by acting apathetic in the spectrum of taking care of Father when he was already approaching his *final* days.

What the strategy Mother now plotted was that she would take care of Father on her own terms.

As for Father, never did he utter a word of blame or gripe about Mother's unwillingness, indifference or inability in taking care of him. He felt grateful every time Mother offered him help instead.

Sam called, telling us not to worry, saying Father was at home lying in bed and talking. Sam described Father as being a bit better than he was at the restaurant, willing to talk, and wanting to watch television. We asked Sam if he had gotten anything to eat, and he said he would cook something available in the kitchen. We thanked him for taking Father back home, saying we would bring him food served from the dinner. Yeah, we are living in a family of love and bonds. Especially, we four siblings love each other very much, and all the time, we see Father as our icon in terms of love.

The next day, we could not wait to go see Father, desperate to see him when the previous night he was so fragile that he failed to have the dinner with us. Father smiled upon seeing us. We could not help giving him our big hugs with tears that we never did in the past. For the Chinese, love is a word that is not as easy to speak out as it is for the Westerners, nor are hugs as easily given. Anyway, all these would be about to *change*. We would hug Father as many times as we could to show him our love, care, and feeling. We knew it was a bit late, but we believed that late is better than never, especially given we felt such hugs were really something so special and important that nothing could replace. The hugs, more than anything, could say how much we loved and missed each other.

We told Father that Christmas was around the corner, and we would have about a week's holiday. We asked him if he had any places he wanted to go to or visit that we could then take him to. Father sweetly replied to us that there was no place like home and no one like us he wanted to be with, distinctly meaning he would be happy enough if we could go home always to be with him more. We could not wait to promise him that, saying we would come home more to play mah-jong with him. He smiled and nodded.

Father appeared a little bit stronger than yesterday despite being a lot weaker than the past few months. It was heartbreaking, though. He insisted he could play mah-jong with us when we asked him to take a rest in bed. Over the mah-jong table, we forced ourselves to concentrate on the fun of the game to attempt to escape any words that would inadvertently come out relevant to Father's illness and destroy the atmosphere we found important amid such a harsh time. It did require us not a little skill in disguise, and we found such disguise we posed had already clandestinely matured into a kind of form we got along with each other—only we could not remember when it started. We talked about some funnier or more popular subjects to create an ambiance of pleasure and delight to gain us happiness that we found precious and necessary since the situation now was so challenging and grim.

Understandably, when a person is badly sick, there should be some space for him to breathe whenever there can be. Merely continually talking about his illness would only pose a great pressure on him that makes him feel more afflicted. Yes, it is true to everyone who is ill—Father no exception.

Father played and played, smiled and nodded regardless of win or loss. He could be easily satisfied not just now being ill but even at the time he had been healthy. He was definitely a man who could give anyone something to learn from him without him literally preaching or teaching but by the others seeing and feeling.

Vomit posed a rather harrowing occurrence to Father when he was now in the stage that his illness was incurable.

Christmas came, meaning we would have holidays, and holidays meant we would come home more frequently than working days. Father was glad about it when he knew he could see us more. Above all, we had to deal with his vomit first. We called Dr Chu, telling him Father's situation. 'Come to my clinic to take some pills. It may help stop the vomiting.' The doctor replied to us over the phone without probing into the reasons why Father vomited. Due to needing it urgently, we did not have other choices but to get the pills the following day. What we hoped was that the pills could stop Father from vomiting so he could eat to stay alive as a fundamental requirement of living. When with such basic requirement fulfilled, he could then talk about quality life.

The following day, we could not wait to take the pills Dr Chu had arranged for us. With the pills on hand, we immediately rushed home to let Father, at the quickest, take it in hopes of being able to eat with it then.

As soon as we got to him with a full plastic bag of pills, Father appeared excited, getting up from the bed and taking a pill down without delay. Not knowing what actually happened to the inner parts of his body, he responded in throwing up not long after taking it. Although it was ridiculous to complain that the pills could not stop vomit with its name interpreting it could do so, we had to hold it up to mockery to vent our indignation. Father kept his head on one side, kept his chin up on the other, saying he would try again later.

The pills were Father's lifeline. When we last night talked about taking it from Dr Chu's clinic, Father appeared more than passionate about it, saying if he could eat without vomiting, he could take care of himself. At least he would not starve to death, he added with a sense of sardonic humour.

Now the pills seemed ineffective. Worse still, it made Father vomit more times. Should we continue to let him try or stop him? We hesitated, not knowing if the pills would further worsen the situation he was in.

As dubious as it could be, all the same, we supported Father in his courage and attempt to take the pills one more time when he said he had to take it once again to prove if it could really work. 'Try, try, and try' is such a popular axiom for encouragement. It seemed, to us, more than a belief at this critical moment. When all of us were in keeping with such a try, Father took it down without second thought.

Much to our chagrin and misgiving, hours later, Father vomited again. In this case, all of us, including Father could not but decide to give the pills up. Asked if Dr Chu had explained the pills to us, John said the doctor told him that the pills he prescribed Father were the ones he usually prescribed to cancer patients to stop or at least ease their vomiting. With this theory, we could not merely find fault with the pills. Judging from Father's situation, we could not but begin to worry that the cancer in him was causing his health to deteriorate. We could only plead that day would not come too soon, and right now, all we could do was to stay with him more and more to make him have the happiest and the most comfortable moments with us that we insisted he deserved.

The pills for vomit failed to work. We furiously set our hands to seek some other pills conducive to Father's poor situation. At last, we found a kind of pill with stronger tonic, which said having the ability to enhance immunity. Another kind was specialized for his liver, which said having the ability to wind down the speed of the cancer from growing fast and fiercely. We just tried this and that in hopes of decelerating any potential worsening inside his body the cancer might cause, with a view to anticipate him not just getting a prolonged life but also living a life with at least the *quality* a human being should have.

Father took the pills we got him and found they seemed to be acting on him with a good response for the time being. With such pills, Father could at least take some food, and with food, he could live, we thought. We just hoped all those pills we got him could make him live and stay with us not only the longest but also the least afflicted.

At dinner, Father took a little rice and soup before holding up a glass of water to cheer with us. Father was more than a considerate person liable to take care of others' feeling in the first place. When we worked so painstakingly to find him this and that with only one wish to make him stay with us, we could feel that he was touched and grateful, many times appearing speechless, with eyes saying thanks to us. When things failed to work, he could feel our hearts break and ask us not to over-worry. The way we used to communicate with Father was so simple and understanding that made us emphatically connected always.

Christmas is welcomed as one of the most jubilant and harmonious festivals for the highest and lowest of all races to celebrate with families, friends, lovers, and whomsoever you want without respect to whether you are a believer or not. With a lot of conspicuous light adornments and buzzing crowds peppering most of the whole world, it is the testament of Christmas deserving a universal festival.

Although without the real Santa Claus's sleigh pulled by reindeers as the old legend said, from Christmas Eve to Boxing Day, it is more than easy to find people spilling onto the streets with laughter and joy, sharing their happiness with their loved and important ones, eating, drinking, chatting, singing, dancing, hugging, exchanging whispers and gifts, and so forth.

As far as our family is concerned, we would avail ourselves of this occasion to share the great and wonderful moment with each other. By showing love and care on one side and on the other playing a role of a little Santa to give away as many gifts as we can, mainly to the younger ones, we have made Christmas a joyous day every year. This year, we would do exactly what we did in the past, attempting to create some special moments distant away from the sad ambiance that set in and held swing lately, in order to let Father and us entering into another kind of ambiance in which we would only feel great.

This year, we were going to buy Father a radio as present after knowing that he wanted a radio in an old model that would only provide channels without any other functions of state-of-the-art that would mess him up. What he meant was he wanted one that was the easiest to operate. Nevertheless, it was once again heartbreaking when we knew there was a hidden truth behind it. It was so he could listen to the radio when he could not sleep at night. 'It is too silent at night,' Father said, sighing. He said some sounds in a dead-silent room might make him feel a bit more secure. Whatever Father said to us, we would say him ayes to support him, and as if by magic, Father, in return, would find himself the most confident with our ayes said to him. Aside from ayes, applause and laughter were all the things we always responded to him as encouragement and consent and mainly understanding. That could explain why we were so connected.

Christmas is a Western festival involving sharing a feast of well-known Western food designated for the day, including the staple: a big fowl called turkey that is always roast. However, we would have food on our own, catering to our taste regardless of the tradition.

Wine, meat, chicken, fish, duck, salads, eggs, vegetables placed the table a spectacular look ever. We all sat down, shoulders touching shoulders, creating a warm and harmonious atmosphere which we always relied on to gain happiness, especially when the time was as tough as the present. Over the table, there were not only delicacies; there was, in effect, laughter dominant—except there were worries and sadness behind it.

Father was so considerate that he stayed out for the dinner with us aiming to make us happy. We thought he must have known we wanted him to do so. He sat mostly at the dinner table, taking a little food once or twice, listening to what we talked about with each other and sometimes responding to us a bit. He seemed immensely reluctant to miss any moment there we were sharing, clinging to every bit of it tightly and happily. The very recent smiles became our most cherished possessions once we got together. On these we relied heavily—not only to make each other happy but also chiefly to hide or flee from sorrow, preventing any one of us from bursting it out, which would stir up an immense sadness that we might not manage. Peremptorily, we were sentimentally forcible-feeble.

Owing to the issue of vomiting Father still had, he could just take a little food each time, and mostly fluid food. Even so, he all the same vomited.

Continuously vomiting, Father appeared weaker and weaker. Still, he smiled and smiled, saying he was all right whenever we asked after him. Father had not asked us about his illness, so we could not know whether he had ever doubted the last operation had successfully removed the new tumour in the anus. In fact, we felt it difficult to tell him the truth, fearful that it would cause him to be further afflicted. The situation with Father now was that there was cancer inside his body occurring majorly to two places that were incurable. Father did not know about it all. Was it good or bad? We only knew it was good to have him live without fear when the time he could have was so limited.

We remembered that Dr Chu had explained to us what he had done in the last operation Father underwent, saying he had reopened the closed artificial excretory opening on one side of Father's abdomen for solid waste excretion. The aim was to make Father decrease the times of excretion through the anus until it stopped. Dr Chu also said Father would have at least six to nine months' quality life, saying we did not have to over-worry. Despite what he said about Father hitting us hard, we accepted the truth and looked forward, hoping we could let Father live the happiest with the least fear or worry.

Lamentably, what was happening to Father now was nowhere near matching what Dr Chu said. The times Father excreted through anus were no less than before with the closed artificial excretory opening reopened. Conceivably, it was torture. That was also the major reason that made Father become fragile and fragile. Besides, he could not eat normally. Every meal, he just took a little food. What was worse, he vomited them out all later on. We, by no means, could agree with such condition as a quality life as Dr Chu promised, even we could barely agreed on the perspectives of medicine over a badly ill octogenarian approaching the stage of his final days.

It was not exactly what we expected to see from Father with the words of Dr Chu. We finally consulted him over the phone.

'I'm sorry that your Father's situation can only be that as you mentioned, for the cancer has already spread not only to one area but possibly the other. There is really so little medicine can do to him when he is in a rather old age. If the case gets worse, you may send him to the hospital to see if there is a softer tack in medicine to soothe his pain. And at this moment, I can only suggest electrical therapy to him to hopefully shrink the size of the tumour the anus develops.' Dr Chu said. Anyway, it would all depend on a number of factors, he added.

In this case, we could only keep an eye on Father's development and do what Dr Chu had suggested us.

Father, a man full of philosophy, enjoyed the essence of life by living harmoniously with everyone he loved and knew. Such was the way he lived that made him earn a very stable and harmonious human relationship throughout his life. Never did he initiate any fight with others, nor did he require anyone to do anything for him. He was a nice and peace-oriented man living in a world where, these days, the messages many convey to one another are so chock-full of utilitarianism.

The most magical way he could get along with everyone well was that he never interpreted what people said to him in another way. He just digested it straightforwardly without thinking if it would carry any connotation bad or negative. The way he communicated with people was a rarity, and such rarity was really special and precious in a world we are living now, full of greed, jealousy, suspicion, and hypocrisy. As the case stands, Father had spoken volumes for the maxim teaching us that virtue is its own reward.

Mother just played her part as a helper in taking care of Father. Never had she showed him much love. However, Father still found it a blessing and chose to believe she always loved him. Such was his great wisdom that had us heap praise and admiration.

On Boxing Day, the second day of Christmas, Father opened the present we gave him. 'Good! An old model, I know how to use this.' Said Father with his signature smile and nod shown. He thereupon brought it back to his bedroom, placing it on a low drawer next to his bed. With our eyes could not help following his *shadow* walking, we were overcome with sadness triggered. Such was the shadow that told us how much he cherished the love he had with us. Such was the shadow that told us how lamentable one day it would be when he would leave us. When we could barely hold our tears, we prayed and prayed, hoping he could live longer and longer, staying with us happier and happier.

At mealtime, Father sat at the table, gazing at the food served. More recently, each dish was like a viewing dish to him when he now, in a sad pickle, could only take less than a little or even none of it. Nevertheless, he chose to sit with us, looking at us eat. 'It is already a pleasant thing to have you all with me at a table,' Father said. 'It matters none if I can eat or not. Anyway, I would get some of the food I want, not to worry.' He said quietly. We ate and chatted as usual to prevent Father from discovering we were sad about him. However flimsy this kind of pretence was, we found it necessary and proper.

The truth was, we were not that afraid of revealing our real feelings to each other, we were just fearful that such real feelings, if revealed, would trigger an outburst of grief, leading to us crying like rainfall and causing Father to heartbreak.

Father vomited several times daily, making his stomach reject anything that he swallowed. Every day was a relentless ordeal in a pattern of repetitive vomit and excretion. Still, Father went on and on, being more than positive and optimistic. Never had he uttered a gripe but confronted it with as much energy as he could have. Such indefatigability was insanely potent to have happened to an octogenarian who had already undergone an operation three times, with one substantial and devastating, in just half a year.

No matter how strong his will was, his body inexorably failed to support it. When there were many times the spirit was willing but the flesh was weak, it was more than laudable with so fragile a body supporting so strong a will. Yeah, what Father told us was that we are no different when we are in the face of adversity, and only those who can grasp the nettle make a difference and influence others.

These few days' unremitting vomit and excessive excretion, culminated in Father barely getting up from the bed. We could only see him suffer but could not help. Certainly, the truth was, it was not only an affliction to him but also to us. When we were there with him, we could still hold him tightly, accompanying him to walk. When we were not there, the situation could be very bad. For the sake of his safety, we decided to persuade him to go to the hospital to see if anything could help.

We called Dr Chu, telling him of the situation Father was in. He suggested Father admit to the hospital to at least get nutrition first to maintain life when he could not even eat, and then for us to think if he could take electrical therapy.

With Dr Chu's suggestion, we comforted Father, saying to him that he could have electrical therapy to make the tumour located in the anus shrink. 'With this cure, you could get better.' We said by way of consolation. Father nodded without querying us why the tumour would still exist when it was supposed to have had removed in the last surgery. It could have been a question raised by him, but he had not asked it. Therefore, we had every reason to believe that Father knew everything happened to him, only he would talk about what we wanted to hear. Other than strong, he was indeed an exceedingly considerate person whom we had no words to thank. With his so decided reply, we arranged him to go to the hospital.

Father had bestowed upon us a lot of his generosity and kindness he inherited, making us, once born, have his unique character that is beneficial and blessed. As for us, we have never wasted what he had given us—such a gift by way of making the best of it to benefit all the people around us. On the surface, Father was an ordinary person living his life in the most ordinary way. As ordinary as he had ever been, deep down, Father was extraordinary, a lot different from many people who are, wittingly or unwittingly, living a world of fights stemming from the derivative of some sorts of dark side of human nature that puts our world somewhat in an upheaval.

Father, a *silent*, *strong* man, after taking months of painstaking effort in recovery, surviving one enormous surgery and two smaller ones, was again going to the hospital, which he described as being without a choice on one side, and on the other, he looked forward to a hope.

Father embodied a mantra of encouraging us never give up before trying, and never making light of the ghost of a hope god grants.

CHAPTER SEVEN

It was New Year's Eve to 2013, when most of the people chose to spill onto the streets with their loved ones to celebrate the festival with tons of joy. Father was spending his first day at the hospital the fourth time. The last time was just twenty days ago, after receiving a surgery to remove the new tumour grown into his anus. He was waiting again for another treatment with hope. Clearly, the last surgery was far from successful without removing the new tumour. Although he insisted that we should happily go out to celebrate on par with others on this jubilant day, we chose to stay with him at the hospital as long as we could to give him support, warmth, and love he deserved.

'I feel much safer to be here,' said Father with a wry smile before making an explanation. 'Mother, every night at about nine, locks her bedroom door for sleeping, leaving me alone in my bedroom and the house and feeling totally helpless. Such helplessness makes me feel like I am on the verge of death.'

'I'm not afraid of death. I'm just afraid of something even worse,' he continued. 'But she is not good in her own health, suffering different kinds of discomfort. She needs rest by sleeping well without interruptions.' He at once found ways to help rationalize or legitimize what Mother did to him.

Apparently, he did not want to have us regret if he would die in a tragic way. Never did Father ever in his life say anything of Mother but this time!

Hearing what Father said, there was an outburst of sadness erupting from us after knowing how hard he was spending every night fearing like that. Luckily, we could keep a grip on ourselves lest the situation should get messy. We had not said anything about Mother but consoled Father, asking him to stay at the hospital until he got good and strong enough to go home to stand on his own feet. Father plucked up his courage, promising to us with a big 'Yes!' Obviously, Father needed encouragement while being in such a sad pickle.

Father and Mother, though, entered in good faith and pledged to cast in with each other's lot in their marriage as many do, but they failed to share a common dream. Father was an easy-going person, resting on his laurels by working hard every day to earn an honest penny, providing us a roof with necessities. He could get along with every one well with his tolerant disposition towards people. Mainly, he was born benevolent with a liberal mind. Never had he quarrelled with anyone even when Mother found fault with him, demanding this and that from him without rhyme or reason.

Woven throughout Mother's life is a complex. Born with a strong character can easily make her speak nineteen to dozen to her loved ones over a small matter or even a trifle, she is nowhere near Father's mentality. What's more, she longed for a far better or even a luxurious life by not agreeing to merely working hard to earn just a living but dreaming of the unrealistic. She always wished of one day becoming a part of the upper crust, and when she found it far from possible, she would find fault with Father, blaming him as incompetent without in earnest, realizing that Father had already done his best and given his best to us.

As to her disposition towards people, she adamantly finds herself always right regardless of getting down to the importance of relationships. Disastrously, such is the self-righteousness that makes her fail to learn that home is a place where love dominates.

The result is that she used to sacrifice everything to win every quarrel she insists she is right and she has to win. To some extent, she is a person lacking philosophy, harmony, wisdom and mainly love.

Father and Mother even cannot be a pair of strange bedfellows, for they have not slept on the same bed for a long time. Mother had not slept with Father long time ago on the grounds of him snoring in his sleep. Having little admiration for Father, Mother, for life, has failed to learn what Father in effect can teach her in the spectrum of relationship and love.

As Father's colon tumour, having undergone an enormous surgery half a year ago, later spread to the anus and now the liver, Dr Chu said there was little or even nothing he could do for him. He suggested that it was not worthy now to take risks in any kind of treatment. He took into consideration Father's weakness and warned us that any kind of treatment would only highly pose an immediate threat on his life with no mercy. Apparently, it was not what he suggested that he could do to Father over the phone, talking to John, before Father's admittance to the hospital.

As the case stood, we all had a meltdown; however, we relished being with Father in the remaining days he would still have. After long deliberation, we decided not to tell Father that brutal truth. Our thought was only if he lived with hope could he have positive thinking, and only when all these favourable elements imbued in his life could he truly live. Life, hope, and positive thinking are of a significant adherence that makes our lives worth living. We could not but deem what we thought more beneficial than detrimental to him and us in every way.

Imaginably, Father was waiting for the electrotherapy suggested by Dr Chu, which he had heard from us before admittance. In fact, before admitting to the hospital, Dr Chu had explained Father's situation to us over the phone. He suggested electrotherapy be undergone at the earliest, making up for the failure of the surgery practiced twenty days ago. Beyond all expectation, he withdrew such a lifeline Father embraced tightly. He explained by way of a medical perspective later to us that Father was too weak and old to undergo such a surgery now.

Luckily, Father only waited but did not ask; and one day, he said to us that Dr Chu told him that his colon was in good shape enough to get rid of any kind of surgery. Actually, that was the result of our asking Dr Chu to help conceal the truth from him as we did. We found that Dr Chu was worth his salt in terms of it a lot more than his cures to Father. He had given us too many false hopes along the way that he had fallen far short of our expectations and hope. Even when the last surgery fell through, he still guaranteed us Father could have at least six to nine months' quality life. However, what happened then to Father was flat out a horse of another colour.

One night in the second week of Father staying at the hospital, when May went see him, he appeared extremely pained, with a repeated urge to vomit. He did his utmost to hide the pain first but eventually failed to do so due to the excruciating pain. He was compelled to say profusely to May that he was in such horrible pain that he needed to vent. Being unable to help totally, May stood by him, suffering too. Watching him swallowing up by the pain, she only could hang in there as if she were in hell.

When my phone rang, I could not wait to pick it up. 'Sister, I went to see Father after school tonight and found him in immense pain,' was the message coming from a voice that sounded like it was crumbling. 'I found myself totally failing in helping him but could only watch him suffer.' The sound seemed to blur with hoarse cries. It was abundantly clear, May was heartbroken to have had witnessed Father to vomit in such a way she found so intolerable that she was driven crazily emotional. 'When I found I could not leave, he asked me to go home to take care of my children and get some rest,' May paused a while and then resumed talking with an even more unmanageable sentiment. 'How could Father love me so much as to ask me to leave when he was suffering an immense pain? How could I leave? Father, I should not have left! It was insane, criminally insane!' May cried and cried. She was falling into an abyss of agony.

Literally, it was harrowing and gut-wrenching. The only thing we could do for each other was to listen first and then comforted.

Unbelievably, after being tortured a whole night, Father again talked to us with humour as before when we went see him the next day, pretending nothing happened the previous night. What we learned from him is that no one can decide you happy or sad except yourself. Sadness in a life is just some passer-by, and they will eventually go away rather than stay and finally give way to happiness even if it is just for a while.

Father's wisdom was that seeing through a lot of torture did not mean you could live with no more of it then; it only meant you could see your loved ones *one more time*. So why be sad instead of happy when you were so lucky and blessed to have time like this? Yeah, we should learn how to see the *calm* between storms and make good use of these in preference rather than let it waste. Moreover, only storms can make the best sailors, we grasped.

No matter how hard he had to suffer, once he was good, Father liked chatting with us and showing us his smile. In the meantime, the happiest thing was watching each other smile when times were as tough as this.

Owing to the medical nutrition tube implanted into a blood vessel in one of his hands on the second day he admitted, which was helping him survive, the vein was appearing a bit overburdened, turning grey and swollen. This morning Father had undergone a transplant surgery to remove the tube from his hand into his neck, into another blood vessel. The doctor who did it to him could not help praise his endurance of the pain. When the tube was on his neck, we gently touched it, trying to feel what he felt, only to find his neck was terribly slim. It could not be slimmer for a human being. Since he had been ill, Father used to put on a scarf round his neck to keep himself warm, and this was the first time we seriously looked at his neck. Father, how much had you suffered to have such a slim neck that it did break our hearts, and how could you suffer so much pain without a word of blame?

After he had long condemned to a bed or once a while to a chair, Father's right foot grew swollen day by day. What we did was, from the word go, make a decision to offer him a foot massage every time we visited him.

With bare hands, out of love and respect, the way we did this was by lifting up the swollen foot gently at first. Subsequently, lightly then heavily in turn, we moved the toes one by one, moving them up and down as if they were dancing a ballet. After this procedure done, we kneaded the sole of the foot in a professional guise of a masseur. Within an hour, we found the foot less swollen as if by magic. To all intents and purposes, Father had never asked for it; the idea was completely ours. Nevertheless, he would smile and get content when we did it to him, and when we finished doing it, he would nod in answer to our job. Surprisingly, the massage had brought about not a little happiness to all of us amid such an ordeal.

Today, the middle part of the month, I went see Father with Tommy, my son.

When they met, Tommy could not stop offering Father nice words that I had never heard before. Every scene was so touching as to embed in my mind that promising I would never forget. One episode was Father affectionately saying to Tommy, 'Your mother loves you dearly, kid. Really, she loves you more than anyone she loves.' Apparently, Father knew not a little of the relationship between Tommy and me, only he had never alluded to it in front of me before. I felt shameful to have him worried about me when he was in a bad way. While I found myself caught napping in such an unexpected scene, I found it more than welcome, however.

A very good listener was always the role Father used to play in the family. All the time, he chose to let us talk and blame. Every house gets an unmentionable story, and we are no exception too. Father adopted a manner of grinning and bearing it every time the family came up against hardship. Whenever we got a problem, we would strain every nerve settling it for the sake of Father, not because he demanded it but because he never and patiently waited. His charisma, which made everybody who knew extol him, led the family to solidarity amid every potential crisis. Additionally, he was born loving home, setting great store by the family admitting of nothing to come before it.

Obligatory as it could be, it was more than touching when Tommy nodded in response to what Father said to him, he looked at me as I looked at him. I heard him say, 'I know, I know,' and he heard me say, 'Yes, yes, my good son.' We both, at full strength, held back the tears glutting our eyes without saying a word. When the expression is overwhelming, words are superfluous. At the same time, Father lay in the bed with his hand softly touching his own head with eyes uncontrollably growing red, saying to us that he was very happy. 'Today, I am very happy'. Father repeated. I could tell he was holding back his tears. My heart broke! I had a feeling that Father might know he would die soon with us making a point of seeing him this way. Rarely had I ever heard Father and my son say something from so deep. Indubitably, we had already deeply struck a sympathetic chord with one another. At that very moment, we three were as one magically. Father, I felt immensely grateful for you, and I could not think of anything to say to thank you except that I love you.

When we were about to leave, Tommy asked Father to get more rest so that he could get recovered enough to go home and make food for us again, adding how he missed the fried chicken wings Father made every time for us. Father promised him this with a smile and nod.

Father, why there was so little time for us to love you? Not until you had been ill did we know you liked talking and needed love. We could have actually loved you a lot more, only that we were too careless. You ought to have deserved more instead of just this little. We could not but blame ourselves for being that foolish and lazy.

Undeniably, we have done so little for Father when he was healthy enough to do whatever he could. We do owe him a lot in terms of love. However, time was too scarce now for us to regret or to waste. Even a second of time waste would be extravagant. Realizing that merely piling on regret would only get us nowhere, we decided to make every minute to come with Father the happiest and the most memorable. This was our mission and top priority.

David, my husband, accompanied me to visit Father. It was a usual Sunday with unusual mood when we went see him. First, I offered Father a massage for his swollen foot as a prelude. Then we talked. Although he appeared the same like before, chatting with us casually with, sometimes, a bit of humour, he talked about something to us out of character all of a sudden.

He asked David when his mother passed away, saying he could not remember it well. David replied to him that it was already twelve years ago. He then sighed, 'Time is flying,' with eyes looking at the ceiling, as if he was thinking. With that, he asked David where she was buried and if we had visited her grave every year. David said since the land then was scanty and expensive, we had her body cremated and stored in a columbarium, and every year, we did perform worship for her. He nodded without further saying anything, even when I asked him what he was thinking at that moment.

Presumably, Father began to be aware that his illness might be incurable and started to feel concern about the undertaking after his death. For a certainty, Father would not easily forget anything. I supposed that he asked it with connotation and hoped that we might read between the lines.

With such an implication from Father, we, on reflection, found ourselves with an obligation to tell him we had bought him a land located in Chaoyang, his homeland, where a litany of memories of his childhood were chronicled in nooks and crannies. This was to be his final place of rest when he would be eternally free from suffering.

The next day, Mother told him about it. She said to him that the land bought was just for future use, and she was sure that he could recover and go home before going there. Obviously, she was elaborately making some humours of it to alleviate the sadness the ambiance held with such a depressing topic. Father said by way of understanding that the cost of the land was modest and the place tranquil to conclude the conversation the soonest, making the unpleasantness the ambiance held vanish into thin air to give free rein to other subjects more pleasant. Wonderfully, Father could effortlessly deal with predicament more than anyone can.

It was the fourth week this month. Father got increasingly weaker. Dr Chu prescribed him some stronger medicine accordingly. A kind of tonic, mainly to alleviate the severe pain occurring constantly over his chest, was started an injection. Father's response was to be relieved not a little as a result. He gradually began to vomit less and less, but at the same time, he lost all the appetite he had and cherished before. Additionally, he was exceptionally tired but could not sleep well. He spent time lying in the bed, sometimes with eyes open to check out who were there to see him. Sometimes his eyes would close so he could take five or think. Seeing him acting this way, we could not think of anything to do but to love him even more. Deep down, we wanted to talk about death to him to see if he had anything to say to us. On second thought, we chose to talk about pleasure to him all the same in order to get his chin up, although we found hearing his last words was no less important than that.

Today, the last Saturday this month, Father appeared unusually talkative. We saw it as a miracle god showered onto us with not a little sympathy we deserved.

Chiefly, Father said to us how much he was eager to go home. He first described to us the typical life of a badly ill patient staying at the hospital. He said his daily struggle was one word: *Wait*. In the morning, waiting for the breakfast he had ordered. At noon, waiting for Mother's food, it is a pot of water like congee, too bland to swallow. In the afternoon, waiting for our turns to see him to give him support and love that he saw as the most lovable moments in a day. In the evening, waiting for the night he feared most. After receiving and confronting all the pains and fears the illness brought all night, he waited for another morning—a new day with no different pattern.

Secondly, he portrayed to us the intensity of the eagerness he had to go home when Chinese New Year drew near. When he was talking about this significant festival, he could not be more excited, looking at all of us with an infinitely broad smile and eyes lighting up. We too were so excited as to see him constructing a beautiful picture of the dinner we would have every time in the New Year. He said he would not only play mah-jong with us, he would make us delicious pastries like every year before as well. We could not but promise him this one by one with a lot of joy and applause. We asked him to stay happy all the time so that he could get better enough to go home. 'Of course' was always the phrase he used to reply to us. That night, we were more than happy to fill the room where silence more often than not reigned over with a lot of laughter and sound.

No matter how ravaged Father's body was, the illness imposed on him could by no means ravage his *mind* a bit. He was more than conscious with as much self-esteem as a normal person

Although it is crazily brutal for a human being to have a conscious mind with self-esteem bearing on a ravaged body constraining one's activities, making one fail in attending to wishes or even basic needs, we would have it that the situation reversed would be the most brutal. We consider that only with a conscious mind can people truly connect with one another with as much love and joy leaving as many unforgettable memories as possible, which make life the most meaningful and adorable. We further decide the point of life is so.

It was the last week this month, a little more than half a month ahead of the Chinese New Year, when Father's condition rapidly deteriorated in a big way. For all that, he was more than conscious. It was such as to render us heartbroken.

Father's old die-hard friends, a very nice and kind couple, came to see him today. Fearful that separation might not be far away, they shook hands with Father and offered him their deepest and most cordial comforts with some unspoken sentiments. Peeping at Father, only to find his eyes red with a slight but perplexing smile, I realized that he must be very hard to find a word to utter. The scene was so sad that I found myself struggling with a pair of eyes full of tears. I could not but demand my feet to run as fast as they could to the washroom, on one hand to prevent Father seeing me cry and on the other to work off some of my long-suppressed emotions.

Father, we really could not know how you hid your tears when it was supposed to flood your eyes. We had seen there were moments you resorted to let it bitterly linger instead of dropping it down. We knew you did it for the sake of our tears, and we knew it was very hard for you. That ability inside you had from time to time amazed us. We had no words to thank you but to love you all out.

Father asked Sam to find him a watch. Since the clock that told him time was located at the front area of the bed, Father found it hard to take a glimpse at it, especially when these past few days he was completely condemned to a bed, unable to lift his body up and to turn his head. "'I want a watch to see the time,'" Sam recounted Father as saying. "'I cannot see the time when I want to. The one located there is hard to see. I sometimes want to see the time even at midnight.'" Sam then brought him a watch with a light, making him able to see the time when the lights were off in the room at midnight. When Sam put the watch over Father's wrist and buckled it properly, Father smiled with much contentment, constantly touching it.

I did not know why I would cry at hearing Sam speak of Father wanting the watch. I just had a feeling that Father was feeling hard, he must have thought the time now was *scarce*— so scarce that he found every minute of it extravagant to him. He must think he had to watch the time lest he should miss one minute. He did not sleep at night in order to save the time, clutching every one of the minutes that he saw would only be less and less. He did not want to let the time pass by. He was now catching up with every minute to see us and let us see him.

Father was an exceedingly nice person, a peace-oriented man. He used to be quiet and somewhat elusive, so we always thought he did not need love. He demanded nothing, nor did he complain about anything. Again, we thought he did not expect it. When, through this half a year, he had lain in the bed suffering pain the illness brought, he began to talk more with us. When he had revealed more of his feelings to us, we had eventually found he was an affectionate man with a lot of sweet and mild paternal love, whose wonderfulness had from time to time amazed us not a little. Nevertheless, we could not but feel so sorry to have had known it so late. Surely, we had not loved him enough before, and we could only feel deep regret about it.

Remarkably, Father started to talk less this week.

Dr Chu called us, explaining the situation Father was in. He said the time might come very soon, and he asked us to make ourselves psychologically prepared. In a matter of days, Father would have to be given morphine. Dr Chu especially warned us that Father could only live in coma for a day or two after he was on morphine, and then he would peacefully pass. He reminded us that if there were words we had yet to say to Father or hear from him, meaning we would have to say now.

At the same time, Dr Chu said that he had asked Father whether he would need the hospital to give him emergency resuscitation at the last moment and got his answer: 'No'. Hearing what Dr Chu said, we were shattered inside out, with all our faces in tatters. After all this, we decided to be undaunted by the awful truth by categorically promising each other once again that we would courageously go through the uphill battle with Father till the last minute, without reservation.

Father—appearing as if small potatoes, a humble and great man in substance—never coveted any bells or whistles but to cherish his four good children. Despite all his life was no adventure, it was a dedication to all his loved ones. Contented with living in obscurity, he worked hard every day to earn an honest penny to provide us a roof with warmth and all the necessities without us worrying. This was his greatest pleasure and satisfaction. He, coming from nowhere, was not lucky enough to have even a modest education but blessed enough to have been born with a lofty integrity that made everyone who knew him place him on a pedestal.

Today, Father did not talk. Instead, he gazed at us longingly, sometimes with a slight smile.

In return, we caressed him gently with love and with light-hearted conversations in order to make him comfortable. We did not talk about death to him, not because it was a depressing subject or even a taboo, but because we found it contrary to our mission. Our mission was to make his remaining scarce and precious times the most comfortable. In a way, we had disregarded what Dr Chu reminded us of earlier. Rightly or wrongly, we promised with each other that we would have no regrets. With not a doubt on our minds, we would only clutch tightly at every minute with Father with only one aim—rendering him as much happiness and ease as possible.

Father was dosed with morphine, he fell into a coma. We stood by him, watching him breathe strenuously with eyes sometimes struggling to open. It was the last day of the month, a Thursday.

At short intervals, the nurses would come to Father in turn, putting a long, slim medical tube inside his mouth, inserting it through the throat to aspirate out of his mouth the harmful phlegm from his lungs, which they said would immediately claim his life if stuck. Oddly enough, Father would use his hands to ward off the nurse's hands during the process. Such a phenomenon was at variance with what Dr Chu had said to us that once father was on morphine, he could only live in a coma and felt nothing. We also had consulted some other nurses' advice over it, and they explained to us that it was merely caused by the reaction of instinct, as a knee-jerk reaction, and was seen as normal. Nevertheless, we were still unconvinced. Instead, we chose to believe what Father presented was a sign of his consciousness, in which he was telling us he knew we were there. At the same time, we have heard not a few times he had made some roars deep from this throat like protesting to us. We saw it as another clear proof.

I was paying full attention every minute the whole day to the electrocardiograph machine, which mainly monitored Father's heartbeats. It was the first time I had seen one ever in my life. Not until this moment did I find seeing it in reality was far more sensational than seeing it in a movie. I fondly wished, ridiculously, that it would give Father a miracle if we befriended it as soon as we knew it. Whenever the curve displaying on the screen indicated that Father's heart was beating, we appeared happy with applause. Whenever it did the contrary by pausing as a straight line, we appeared sombre.

Father was great enough to fight tooth and nail to inhale at every critical moment. Presumably, he did not want to leave us when he knew we were there with him. Yeah, it was hard—insanely hard—for Father and all of us.

This morning, we rushed to the hospital to see Father after being informed that he was near death.

When we arrived, the nurses was attending to Father, they explained to us that he could barely breathe when some phlegm was stuck his throat. Luckily, the phlegm was in time aspirated out. Seeing Father again breathe, we relieved not a little. Conceivably, it was a matter of course that Father would pass away in a matter of days, so why would we still live in hope that he would live, were we living in dreams reluctant to wake up to face the truth? Such a thought was so crazy that it could only be *inexplicable*. Yeah, we were living in fantasy. Human beings are the most sentimental creature may serve us an answer to it.

No matter how much we did not want to eat, Mother urged us to take some food. Therefore, we favoured her by taking our lunch downstairs in turns, at the hospital's canteen, to remain energetic enough to come back to stand by Father.

Pathetically, we dared not admit that we were waiting for Father's last moment to come when we dared to look at that monster-like machine. Life could not be any worse or more sarcastic in facing such a tormenting predicament.

Concededly, life has us learn that we are living in a cauldron of happiness and sadness in which no one can filter out the good and throw out the bad. They are bound to intertwine. Life, as well, feeds us abundantly a cauldron of philosophy, in which 'There is a time for everything' tells its own tale. To be plain or more precise, life and death is a journey wherein everyone just needs to take their course. At this rate, the laws of life can lead myriads of creatures on earth to pass on normally and orderly.

Today, the second day of February, eight days ahead of the Chinese New Year, we were by Father's side loyally with love.

Father appeared markedly weaker than the past two days although he still breathed. Notably, the breaths he took were far weaker than before, and we could tell how the situation was from the extent of the paleness of his face. More than clearly, he could not be any frailer. Once a burly man—as sound as a bell, with the image still fresh on our minds—he had been ruthlessly turned into a bag of bones after going beyond skinny to skeleton while now waiting for his last moment. Brutally, it had unscrupulously turned all our hearts upside down.

Rather than sat on the thorns, we stood by Father all the time, holding his hands and talking to him. He was aware of our existence, we insisted. In the light of this insistence, we did not say goodbye to him despite us finding it a responsibility or a must—we were still hoping for a miracle.

Mom again urged us to take something to eat to maintain our energy. She said we could not do anything well afterwards if we lacked good health. What she said was so self-evident that it needed little explanation. Hence, we immediately took our turns going to the canteen as quickly as we could in response to her good will and request. Deep down, in extreme fear of missing Father's last breath, none of us wanted to leave him *for a minute*.

Father again strenuously inhaled after pausing for some seconds every time. Such a phenomenon happened several times, and each time was like killing us. We knew the moment drew near—so near that we sometimes dared not even breathe to attempt escaping the fright.

Likely, there was a sign we knew the moment was coming. It was something only people of one flesh and blood, people sharing the same pulse, could sense.

It was *second of February; the time, ten minutes past two.* All of a sudden, the room burst into a roar of wailing. Truly, Father was gone. The cruellest reality eventually appeared in front of our eyes. He could not inhale anymore. He had finished all his breaths, with each one more strenuous than the last. He went after being all out to do us a great favour. We concluded that he went with the most esteem to complete his life by fully fulfilling his obligation in terms of cradle to grave. He was our *father,* a *hero* as well as our *exemplar.*

At that very moment, we could not think of anything but to wail uncontrollably. When we buried our broken faces into each other's shoulder to drown the sorrow in grief insanely, we found what we felt was not only sadness or helplessness but also security and love. Most importantly, that security and love were so strong and intimate that they had broken through some of our grief drown. When we were pouring out the grief, at the same time, we had not forgotten to take care of each other's feelings by offering consolations to the one who leant on. Really, Father had a magic to make us converge in every way.

Not until this moment were we willing to say 'Father, *goodbye.*'

'Dad, may you rest in peace. Let us join you one day. Remember that you have never been alone, for we are with you always. Thank you for the very strength you have exercised all the time when you could not afford to let us see you, especially the last three days. You are more than great over it, and we cannot find a word competent enough to show you our gratitude.

'Dad, you will never know how much we want to tell you the following: the way you respect life has taught us a valuable lesson that will be so influential to our lives afterwards. The way you thrive in adversity has afforded us a precious experience that we can in no case gain elsewhere, and the way you managed to make the unbearable bearable when life has you dance to its tune has taken our breath away. Literally, you have thrilled us from time to time.

'Although from the day you started receiving cure to this moment is so short that we will see it as unfair and ridiculous, we are not going to put blame over it, since we find our efforts have been paid off. Such is the pay-off: it has made us believe that life is eventually worth living no matter how short. Such is the pay-off: it has made us learn that we should take nothing for granted and we should always feel blessed. Such is the pay-off: it has made us discover that life is not only meaningful but also beautiful. Such is the pay-off: it has made us fully realize that how much you really mean to us. Most importantly, such is the pay-off: it has made us know what a father you are to us though we have known so *little* of you before.

'You have brought up in the world four decent persons with your integrity and love. You have spoken great volumes for how example is better than precept. What you have left us is something of such far more meaning and benefit than a great fortune that we will bring it into full play in our lives to benefit others as you always do.

'Although we failed to keep our words to bring you home, we pledge we will one day all be together somewhere we belong, to again share our happiness and love. Goodbye, our sweet beloved dad.' We said to Father round his bed, almost in unison, as if we had rehearsed it before.

Later, a doctor came to Father, mainly to that machine, to note down the time of death. 'Certified,' the doctor said. We knew it was time to let Father go peacefully. We stopped crying but gave him our goodbyes with our sweetest smiles instead.

The past half a year and this very moment—long because they were bitter, short because they were sweet—collected all the bitterest and sweetest memories of Father and us. All of these memories cohere sweetly and bitterly, and we are not going to select any of those to remember but to remember them as one always for life.

To such a silent, strong man as you have ever been, Father, however much we have said to you, words are inadequate or incompetent anyhow. We would only have you know that we have found you the *best* thing in our lives, and we promise that we will love you and remember you forever and a day in our hearts.